"As a pharmacist, I see and hear the frustrations of mental health and addictions clients every day. The unique and innovative approach in this book could serve as a template, not only for this field, but for improving the delivery of many areas of health care in Canada."

—Jack Davies, Pharmacist

"In my 32-year career as a registered nurse, I have not seen any approach that is as simple, innovative, and fundamentally important to the mental health and addiction field, as the ideas presented in *It's Not About Us*. This is a must-read for all nurses."

—Marguerite MacDonald

"Clinicians should not be afraid to adopt this model of service delivery as it will enhance not only their clients' experience of the service, but enable them to deliver client-centered treatment in the manner for which they were trained.".

—Dr. Andrew Ashley-Smith, Psychiatrist

"This piece of work should be a blueprint guide for health change leaders in Canada"

—Kevin Fraser, RSW, RCC, manager - mental health and addictions.

IT'S NOT ABOUT

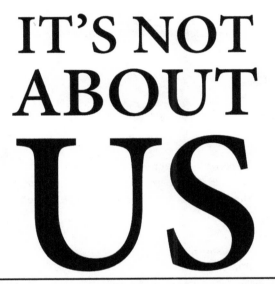

US

The Secret to Transforming the Mental Health
and Addiction System in Canada

TODD LEADER

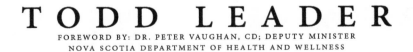

FOREWORD BY: DR. PETER VAUGHAN, CD; DEPUTY MINISTER
NOVA SCOTIA DEPARTMENT OF HEALTH AND WELLNESS

Editor: Hubert E. Devine

Library and Archives Canada Cataloguing in Publication

Leader, Todd, author
    It's not about us : the secret to transforming the mental health
and addiction system in Canada / Todd Leader ; foreword by Dr. Peter
Vaughan, CD, Deputy Minister, Nova Scotia Department of Health and
Wellness. -- First edition.

Includes bibliographical references.
Issued in print and electronic formats.
ISBN 978-0-9938173-3-5 (paperback).--ISBN 978-0-9938173-2-8 (HTML)

    1. Mental health services--Canada. 2. Substance abuse--Treatment--
Canada. I. Title.

RA790.7.C3L39 2016   362.20971   C2016-906160-4
                                               C2016-906161-2

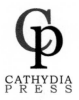

CATHYDIA
PRESS

www.cathydiapress.ca

Print Book - 978-0-9938173-3-5
E-Book - 970-0-9938173-2-8

This book is dedicated to those of you who have experienced challenges with addiction or mental health issues, and have struggled to obtain the kind of support you needed...when you needed it, and also to those whom I hope in future will be able to benefit from a system that is transformed to become client-centered.

TABLE OF CONTENTS

FOREWORD

Todd Leader's prescription for mental health services in Canada is timely. Todd has the benefit of experience on the frontlines in Nova Scotia where he led the change in service delivery to a model that focused on the needs of individual patients and their families over the interests of how providers want to organize services for their own convenience. Easy to say, hard to do. In this book Todd charts a path for policymakers and clinicians alike and he challenges all of us to think differently about how mental health services could be organized if we put ourselves in the place of those individuals seeking our care.

So, it turns out the secret to transforming care is no secret at all, it's really better customer service. Actions and redesigned services that actually put people first is a major culture shift, one that is currently being enabled by the rapid uptake of digital health technology, a major shift that promises to democratize health care the way the Gutenberg Bible changed the face of religious culture. To operationalize the changes Todd envisions, to see that the phenomenology of client-centered care is in your hands, or your mobile device, will allow all of us to create better access to mental health services than we could have imaged if we remain tethered to the past, the way things have always been done.

The concept of client-centered care is not new. It exists as a principle claimed by all health care organizations. What is new about this book is that it provides us an approach to turn a principle into transformation, which has always been the most elusive part. By applying an approach that is not inherently clinical but is about systems instead, and by doing so from a client perspective, this book enhances our ability to move beyond the words and into action. Todd Leader has implemented change, and he's asking us to join him in creating the future we want to see for better, more timely access to mental health and addiction services.

Dr. Peter Vaughan, CD

Deputy Minister, Department of Health and Wellness

Nova Scotia

PREFACE

Is There a Problem with The Mental Health and Addiction System in Canada?

Virtually every day or week across Canada, the media report stories that answer this question loud and clear. Look closely and you will find such stories extending over many years. They present some diversity of concerns, but they all share some common themes. People do not feel that the system responds to their needs, treats them as important, or understands their unique perspectives and experiences as persons dealing with mental illness. They do not feel the leadership of the system puts their needs above other issues of bureaucracy, politics, finances, or efficiency. I have selected some headlines from across the country to provide a snapshot of this national picture, from the client/public perspective.

"**Mental health services harder to reach in Nova Scotia**" (The Chronicle Herald, Nova Scotia, 2016)

"**Discharged: Mental health patients raise alarms about care in Winnipeg**" (Jill Coubrough, CBC News Manitoba, 2013)

"**B.C. mental health system failing teens, watchdog says**" (CBC News, British Columbia, 2013)

"**Yellowknife LGBTQ community wants more inclusive health care system**" (Shannon Scott, CBC News, 2016)

"**N.S. woman struggling to find mental health services for friend in need**" (Kayla Hounsell, CTV Atlantic News, 2016)

"**Mental health system failing, says Calgary widow**" (CBC News, Alberta, 2010)

"**Canada's mental health system is failing children in crisis**" (University of Waterloo, School of Public Health and Health Systems)

"**Critical gaps exist in mental health services in P.E.I. for vulnerable children, youth**" (Teresa Wright and Doug Gallant, The Guardian, 2016)

"**We are failing young Canadians on mental health**" (Michael Kirby, The Toronto Star, 2013)

"**Mental health review will show fragmented system, failures to act on previous recommendations: Swann**" (Darcy Henton, Calgary Herald, 2015)

"**Sask. mom wants quicker access to mental health consultant after son dies from fentanyl overdose**" (Devon Heroux, CBC News Saskatoon, 2016)

"**Case exposes failings of mental health system: lawyer**" (CBC News, Newfoundland & Labrador, 2014)

"**Young people often forced to seek help for mental health issues at ER, study says**" (Sheryl Ubelacker-The Canadian Press, CBC News, Toronto, 2016)

"**Wait times for mental health referrals longest in central N.B.**" (Colleen Kitts-Goguen, CBC News New Brunswick, 2015)

"**Mental-health help for youth needs radical reform, says advocate Tony Boeckh**" (CBC News, Montreal, 2014)

"**Ross River, Yukon, residents desperate for mental health services**" (Nancy Thompson, CBC News – North, 2016)

"**Suicide study reveals depth of Nunavut's mental health problems**" (Bob Weber, Canadian Press – Iqaluit, Nunavut; The Globe and Mail, 2013)

"Ontario youth wait a year or more for mental health care: report" (Laura Armstrong, The Toronto Star, 2015)

"Winnipeg mom calling for change in Manitoba's mental health system" (Talia Ricci, Global News Manitoba, 2016)

"Cape Breton mother wants mental health inquiry after son's death" (Yvonne LeBlanc-Smith, CBC News Nova Scotia, 2015)

"Province urged to act on Prince Edward Island mental health crisis" (Jim Day, The Guardian, 2014)

"N.W.T.'s mental health care system failed our son, say grieving parents" (Hilary Bird, CBC News, 2015)

This is just a sample of hundreds of similar headlines available. It doesn't take much analysis to see that across Canada we have a problem with the organization and delivery of mental health services. It is apparent that many people do not feel as though the system can or does meet their needs. Their problems are permitted to escalate to a crisis point, when they really needed help earlier. People repeatedly express their frustration with what they perceive to be administrative and bureaucratic barriers that get in the way of their receiving the care they need. They feel unheard. They feel fear if a family member or friend does not receive help when it is needed. They feel anger if the well-being of their loved one gets worse because of waiting. They feel sadness watching people suffer, while perceiving that suffering to be avoidable. We all watch the news and see these stories on almost a daily basis. It is time for a fundamental change.

Who am I and why am I writing this book?

I have spent the last 25 years working in the public sector in leadership roles. I have led programs and departments which have included mental health, addictions, primary health care, health promotion, community engagement, and chronic disease management. I have also taught many of these content areas in the Faculty of Science at Saint Mary's

University for the same 25+ years, with a specialty focus on leading system change, social change, and improvement of health and social outcomes. As both a Registered Community Psychologist and Registered Social Worker, my perspective has always included a recognition of the need to address individual and population-level needs simultaneously, and also to concurrently address all levels of prevention and treatment.

In 2005, an addiction program under my management was granted two International Best Practices Awards by the Ontario Hospital Association at its annual conference. The primary reason for this recognition was the fact that services were designed and implemented explicitly to meet the clients' needs. Access was made so much easier and more convenient that the number of people getting help increased dramatically (in some cases the number more than tripled). Since that time, I have continued to use similar methods, refining them constantly, to improve client experiences and outcomes.

In 2010, while working at the executive level of Nova Scotia's South Shore District Health Authority, I had the opportunity to restructure and then assume leadership of the newly integrated Addiction and Mental Health Program as part of my portfolio. From 2010 to 2014, our team applied this client-centered approach to the program, in which we focused on the clients' needs in a different way than usual. The results were remarkable – we reduced and in some cases eliminated wait times, improved access to services, and increased public and client satisfaction. This confirmed for our team that there was a *better* way to do things – an approach that could transform the mental health and addiction system and make it work better for the public it is intended to serve. There was, we came to understand, a more effective way to view the system, to actually bring about the transformation that is so clearly needed.

This book is obviously derived in part from a true success story. It is an analysis of the transformational work done by a passionate, talented, and evolving group of leaders and staff in one district health authority in Nova Scotia. The team of people, from front line staff to the CEO, figured out how to design and implement a more responsive mental health and addiction program. They did not become paralyzed by endless planning, and did not become restricted by, or inflexibly caught in, a pre-packaged and structured model of service. Instead, they set out collectively to create the most responsive and client-centered services possible. This involved a number of specific approaches that became the cornerstones of the change. Some of these lessons represent concrete observable actions, while others fall more in the conceptual areas of principles, approaches to leadership, and perhaps even ways of being.

When we began transforming and redesigning the services, we started by setting this concept of client-centered systems and processes as our primary guiding principle. I wanted staff to feel proud, not ashamed, of the program for which they worked. I committed to them that if we truly worked together toward this client-centered system, the day would come when they would be driving home from work and hear a news item that praised the program for a change, instead of criticizing it. I suggested they would read the newspaper or watch television and see positive stories about the mental health and addiction services they offered. They would have clients who were satisfied with the responsiveness of the program and with the way services made them feel. The staff already had many clients who were satisfied with the clinical work that took place behind closed doors, but who also noted that the path to get in and out of that clinical work was often fraught with many frustrations and negative experiences for the client.

That was to be our target. We planned to overhaul the *system* to be client-centered. For the record, in as little as 18 to 24 months later, the negative media reports stopped and we began getting positive news stories about the improvements. In my last two years with that organization, and up to the time of writing of this book, we had no negative media stories regarding our services. Instead, we had many positive print, radio, and even national television stories reported. This was a solid indication that we had successfully attained an unprecedented level of client and public satisfaction. A few examples:

"Health services expand at South Shore schools" (Keith Corcoran, Lighthouse Now, 2012)

"**South Shore students' mental health wait times cut**" (Beverley Ware, The Chronicle Herald, 2014)

"**South Shore wait times slashed; Mental Health, addiction services take 4 weeks instead of 8 months**" (Beverley Ware, The Chronicle Herald, 2013)

"**Big gains for mental health in South Shore; Wait times for mental health services in the South Shore are among the best in the province.**" (Michael Lee, Lighthouse Now, 2016)

"**Wait times reduced by months for mental health, addictions help**" (Stacey Colwell, Lighthouse Now, 2013)

"**Student access to health services shows dramatic improvement**" (Stacey Colwell, Lighthouse Now, 2014)

It is clear to me that none of the individual steps or processes described in this book could themselves have caused the extent of change that was achieved. It is also clear that these changes could not have been achieved without a truly collective approach among a great number of people at all levels of the organization. It was in this context that change was made. Here are some of the compelling highlights:

The Addiction and Mental Health Program achieved a reduction in wait times from eight months for adults seeking outpatient/community-based service down to three to four weeks. This program also achieved a reduction in wait time for children and adolescents from a five-month average down to children waiting only three weeks and regular, non-urgent adolescents getting access in an astonishing one to seven days. These results were then sustained for the two to three years up to the time of writing this book, despite regular fluctuations in numbers of clients or in staff vacancies or absences. During this same time, we also saw seven times more adolescents per year.

As a point of reference, I note that, at the time of writing this book, the published wait times for the rest of Nova Scotia are listed as high as 253 days for adults (Sydney), with many other areas showing upward trends from 2013-2015. For children and adolescents, at the time of writing this book, the published provincial average wait time is 109 days, with a high of 152 days at the Izaak Walton Killam (IWK) Health Centre (the children's hospital responsible for all outpatient adolescent mental health and addiction services in the Central Zone of the Nova Scotia Health Authority).

How did this program do it, you might ask? Well, for that you will have to read the rest of the book. However, I will give you a hint. The answer lies in introducing the concept of a client-centered system. Sounds simple, and it sounds like what everyone already believes they do, right? In my observation, however, an authentic understanding and application of the concept is rare in this field. Conceptually, it may be pretty simple, but it requires meticulous work to actually achieve – perhaps not so much rocket science as brain surgery.

Around the same time as our innovative transformation was occurring, some programs around Nova Scotia began adopting a pre-packaged program model, known as the Choice and Partnership Approach – CAPA (Kingsbury & York, 2013), as a step-by-step guide to accomplish some of the same results we had achieved. For some, the CAPA model began to improve wait times, and began to eliminate some of the old system-centered traditions. However, any such model is limited in its ability to produce the complete paradigm shift discussed in this book. That is why, even in some of the areas that adopted CAPA, unacceptable wait times still exist, and client/public dissatisfaction continues to be expressed in the media. Incidentally, in the south shore area, after achieving many of our transformational goals, we also then adopted CAPA as part of a provincial directive. It did not have any impact on our wait times, which our client-centered approach had already improved more significantly than CAPA did elsewhere. It did, however, provide some useful methodology for the ongoing management of efficiency and equity in caseloads and staff productivity. It also provided some new language that helped support, but did not by itself create, a fully client-centered system.

Having studied and taught these principles and approaches as an academic, while also applying them to our public services in leadership roles, the answers gradually became clearer with every day and year. As I experimented, evaluated, and adjusted the approach, programs improved, access improved, satisfaction improved, media attention improved. My analysis of both the academic and applied portions of this work led me to one primary truth – our mental health and addiction system was not and is not designed to be client-centered, and, when we do make the shift to design it that way, it works better.

The challenge is that I am not talking about tweaking a specific process, adding more staff, improving clinical skills, or adopting a structured model. I am talking about making a paradigm shift. Essentially, that means conceptualizing and designing a new framework into which all our program and service decisions would fit. I am talking about viewing the problem through a different lens, or seeing it from a completely different perspective than we have in the past. Analogously, it is not like changing one's word processing software or the person using it. It's like replacing the operating system. It is not like just eating more of something or less of something, but is about changing how you see your life and where and how food fits into it.

In the past, mental illness was viewed from a paranormal perspective; that is, those who were ill were seen to be witches or as possessed by demons. As we eventually learned more about neurology, biology, and psychology, we stopped interpreting things that way. We instead viewed these issues as being medical or psychological in nature, not spiritual or demonic. That was a major paradigm shift. We redefined the way we interpreted and understood the issue, and thereby shifted from burning at the stake to medication and psychotherapy.

In this book, I am suggesting a similar shift in our model. I am suggesting that – based on a combination of experiential and empirical learning, and an analysis of the past, current, and potential future states of the mental health and addiction field – a move to a client-centered paradigm is necessary. As I will explain, this does not mean we abandon all our current methods and skills, but, instead, we embed them in a new model of assumptions, beliefs, and priorities, and a new approach to system design, service delivery, and operational decision-making. In other words, we embed them in a client-centered paradigm. This book is an attempt to take the success that has been achieved in transforming a mental health and addiction program, and translate that into principle-based actions that can be used more widely across Canada.

INTRODUCTION

About the title

The title of the book conveys two very distinct and important messages:

1 – A common client perception – The title is intended to reflect the perspective and feelings of many who have struggled as clients in the system, or as friends and family members supporting someone with mental health challenges. Time and time again clients and families complain, "It's not about us!" People use many different phrases and words to express this, and always with great emotion and frustration. The common theme is people feeling and observing that the system is not designed around their needs or improving their client experience. They instead perceive it to be designed to meet administrative, financial, bureaucratic, or political needs, or perhaps to meet the personal preferences or rigidity of the managers or staff. Many clients and family members will also say they have been greeted and helped by some nice people along the way who genuinely care. That, however, does little to eliminate the frequent client perception that the *system* is not designed to be *about them*. So, currently and historically, the experience and belief of many clients and their supporters who interact with the mental health and addiction system is *"It's not about us!"*

2 – A core principle to lead system transformation – This title is also meant to be the most important statement of principle to help leaders, managers, and staff in the mental health and addiction system transform it into being truly client-centered. For those designing and operating services, this is a way of viewing your everyday work. In every decision, action, policy, procedure, negotiation, meeting, etc., please be guided by the reminder that it's not about the staff, managers, directors, or politicians. It is supposed to be about the client. Making that distinction is crucial if we ever expect to truly transform and improve the system. So, if you work in the mental health and addiction system, especially in a leadership role, *please* adopt this as your mantra. Remind yourself every day that *"It's not about us!"*, it's about the client.

Purpose of this book

The mental health and addiction field has struggled for some time to meet the demands of the public and the needs of the communities and individuals it is mandated to serve. This is despite the fact that many intelligent and well-intentioned people have been providing the services and providing the management and leadership of the programs. So, what's wrong? Why is it that we can't seem to get it right? Why is it that whenever the mental health and addiction component of our health care system is mentioned in the media, it is most often in a derogatory sense? It is also likely that in many such stories, the frustrations raised will relate to either access to the system, or the experience a client has had within the system.

Changes *are* made. People in the system do try to make improvements. For example, sometimes in an attempt to improve the program, managers and leaders will adopt a pre-packaged model, and a manual is followed step by step until the new process or approach is in place. While such adoption of established models has some value, it typically makes a limited contribution because it is missing some very essential features of leadership, including creativity, flexibility, adaptability, and client-centeredness.

People who have been in public service (or have been watching it from the outside) may also have observed that sometimes things fail to change because of *planning paralysis*. This means that the leaders or managers put so much effort into trying to schedule and map out every step, get it planned perfectly, and foresee every hurdle, that very little is ever changed at a level that actually affects the client.

Sometimes, we also see leaders in the system focus their efforts on their own preferred issues, which may involve creating manuals and training programs that either have a one-time impact, or begin collecting dust without any real change. This may benefit or have an effect on staff, but rarely has an impact on the experience of the client.

As with this tendency to over-plan, to adopt rigid program models, or to focus on personal and professional preferences, there are many other common habits, historical bits of context, or leadership and management styles that commonly keep the client experience from improving. Leaders in these programs need to learn to focus the system on the clients from more of a phenomenological perspective. That really means trying to understand the distinctness of clients' perceptions and experiences, as compared to those of staff and management. It means seeing services through the eyes of someone in need of help, or understanding the way a family feels when advocating for their loved one in need. System leaders need to put aside tradition, history, preferences, professional biases, and extended planning, and start to take truly-committed action toward client-centered processes. This book is about *doing*, and promotes the minimum amount of talking and planning needed in order to get to the *doing*.

Since it is about *doing*, this book is obviously not intended to be theoretical. It is also not intended to be a new model that people can blindly implement and expect the problems in the system to disappear. That would be completely counter to what I have learned and come to believe about effectively leading system transformation through the development of a client-centered approach. As noted already, pre-packaged models often fail to allow for reality to happen, and inhibit the kind of responsive and creative leadership needed for significant change. It is not recommended, therefore, that this book be interpreted as such a model. If it is, we will just end up with more people trying to simply follow a road map, or a step-by-step recipe.

I realize following such a step-by-step process is a legitimate function of management, and is the primary tool of many in management jobs. But, for *transformation* to take place, that cannot be the primary approach or skill set. That is not what is most needed. Rather, I recommend that those in the system explore, discuss, and internalize the principles and concepts described in this book, then use them to lead creatively. Use them to get off any traditional, predetermined, or pre-packaged path your program is on, and instead focus on leading dynamically, flexibly, and incrementally toward client-centered services.

If you are a person who has experienced some of the problems with the current system, as a client or supporter, but perhaps have never really known *how* to help fix those problems, this is your chance. Many people may have had the experience of advocating for change. You may have filed complaints with a local program. You may have written to an elected official or top administrator. You may have gone to the media to tell a story about why the system needs to change. In most such cases, advocates like you do a great job of helping people see what is wrong, and making them believe that it needs to change. Then, it is left in the hands of those in control to figure out *how* to fix it.

Regrettably, the *"how"* has been and remains a major impediment to change. If those same people you advocated with have been the leaders of a program for more than a few years, and the system has not really changed for the client, it is safe to assume those leaders don't really know *how* to bring about change. As an advocate, you can now take the concepts and principles in this book, and go discuss and promote them with the people who run or can influence your local mental health and addiction programs and services. You no longer need simply to ask for it to be improved. If the content of this book makes sense to you as a step in the right direction, you will be better prepared to suggest *how* to make improvements and bring about the needed change. Good leaders will always welcome a discussion with clients and community members about solutions and improvements. So, take this information and engage the leaders and the public in the conversation about making the system client-centered.

CHAPTER 1

WHAT IS A "CLIENT-CENTERED SYSTEM"?

Client-centeredness of a *system* is not just the regular showing of compassion by a health care provider to a patient/client. Rather, it also needs to become the new paradigm that structures all the design and operations of the mental health and addiction system. This chapter will break down the expression "client-centered system" and explore the meaning and intention of its three component concepts, from biggest to smallest – defining and understanding system, then centered, then client. Taken together, they establish the foundation of all subsequent chapters, and provide a way to achieve much of what we want and need our public mental health and addiction programs to be.

"System"

What is a system? It is a collection of parts that are connected, compatible with one another, interdependent, predictable, and that function together for a common goal or purpose. There are social systems like families and communities. They have members who each play predictable roles in relation to one another, keeping relationships and interactions normal and stable. For instance, a child often knows from past experience which sibling, parent, or guardian to go to if he is potentially in trouble, or which to go to for permission to do something, or which to ask for money. There are physical or mechanical systems, such as the engine of a car. Every part was designed specifically to fit together and function well in relation to every other part, in order to create transportation. You couldn't just plug in parts that are incompatible and expect the system to function. The car runs because every part was designed with a single goal in mind. The car runs because the parts were not designed to function independently, but, rather, to work interdependently, in an integrated fashion – as a *system*.

Our mental health and addiction *system* is the set of parts, and normative and predictable processes, behaviours, and interactions on which its programs operate. It has many parts. It includes each employee, each team (i.e., intake, clerical, clinical, community support, inpatient nursing, psychiatry). Each of those parts interacts with many of the other parts on a regular basis to achieve a common purpose, which is to provide service to clients. Those interactions are predictable and compatible with one another. A clinician does not get a new client to work with unless an intake worker gets a call and completes the process of making that person a client. Reciprocally, an intake worker is unable to take in a new client and book him for an appointment until a clinician is able to help another client reach her goals, close the case, and free up a time slot for someone new. A nurse on a unit cannot give medication to a patient unless a psychiatrist has ordered it, and a psychiatrist often cannot order it unless the nurses share their observations of the patient's condition from shift to shift with the psychiatrist.

"Centered"

We all use the word, but what does it mean? We talk about our lives being centered around our children or family. We talk about wanting to feel centered. We talk about our work or services being centered around the people we serve or care for. We may say someone is the center of our universe. When we say something is at the center, we typically mean everything else revolves around it, sometimes literally. The sun is the center of the solar system. The other planets never stray from their paths around it. We have community centers, especially in small rural areas, that truly are the hub of the community. Everything that goes on happens there, like adult dances, children's fun activities, community planning processes, religious events.

In decision-making, the same concept applies. If, for instance, you say your children are the center of your life, that would imply that your decisions and actions revolve around what is best for them. One might also say they are your *priority*. This is a concept at the very core of client-centeredness. Unfortunately, it is one that is taken for granted and rarely explored, but needs to be fully understood.

"Priority" – The Essence of the Word Centered

Many people often use the word *priority* as if it is synonymous with the word *important*. It isn't. The root of the word is prior. The word priority is a term of relativity. It is meant to indicate that one thing comes *prior to,* or *before*, something else.. It is entirely about ranking of relative principles, actions, or perhaps people's needs.

Let's consider some examples. Imagine you are short on cash, and there are two things you need to buy at the grocery store on your way home. Your partner at home, who asked you to stop and get them, indicates that both items are a priority. That doesn't help you at all. It provides no direction to guide your next move. Simply saying they are both priorities does not indicate relativity, and therefore is a misuse of the word. Hence, it will likely get you into trouble no matter what you decide when you get to the store. What is needed is for your partner to use the term accurately and tell you which of the two items is *the* priority over the other. That way, you know which of the two items is *more* important to buy. If you don't have the money for both, you know which to bring home. Certainly, it is possible that both items are needed in order to make dinner. That would mean they have equal priority. However, having that information would also help you because it would direct you *not to buy either item* because neither has any value without the other. But, be clear, if you or your partner end up choosing to buy one of the products, you have made a choice about priority, and in fact they are *not* equal.

Health care leaders and managers face decisions every day that require an understanding of this concept. But, as many likely know, either from honest self-reflection or years of observing others, there is not always consistent adherence to this way of using the term. Far too often, someone gives direction that indicates what "the priorities" are, along with the expectation that people are to address them. That use of the word is relatively uninformative to anyone's decision-making. It merely identifies a collection of things that are important. What people need more often is for that collection to be put in the form of a ranked list, or even a more complex way of understanding the comparative value of the items in that collection.

If we want our mental health and addiction system to be client-centered, that implies that we want our clients to be *the* priority… not *a* priority. It implies that, whenever we look at any component of a program or service, we consider if it is what is best for the client. It means that when facing a choice between two or more important factors, the client's experience and well-being will be automatically considered most important.

Without a clear understanding of the word priority, and the commitment and ability to apply that understanding in everyday decisions, decision-making would be paralyzed or would vary to the point of dysfunction. Throughout this book, the word *priority* will be used quite often. It is a fundamental building block for achieving a new kind of client-centered system, and one that contributes big things to effective transformation.

Client-Centeredness of Systems Rather Than Individuals

For many people working in helping professions, the term client-centered usually elicits thoughts of the work that people do at the individual treatment level. Health care professionals provide compassionate and empathic care as an almost-natural part of how they approach their clients/patients. This caring is commonly thought of and referred to as client-centered.

In the mental health and addiction branch of health care, the term often elicits thoughts of Carl Rogers and his ideas about individual therapy and the factors that create a healthy therapeutic climate (genuineness, empathy, and unconditional positive regard). There is no doubt that, at the individual client/patient level, staff care about their clients' well-being and work to create such conditions. However, the general concept of *client-centered* also needs to be applied at the level of process, policy, and system.

Client-centeredness is not just about how the individual pieces of the system (staff members) do their work. In a system, there are other factors that matter. For example, if we are relying on the level of individual treatment to represent and deliver this idea of client-centered service, then we are going to experience a great deal of variability because of the personality and skill differences among staff. Some clients will feel valued and helped, and others will not. Obviously, some level or type of consistency of approach among those staff is important to ensure all clients have a positive experience, regardless of with whom they interact.

Achieving such consistency is a system issue. It is about hiring the right people, setting policy, listening closely to clients about their experiences, empowering and setting clear expectations for staff, and monitoring and enforcing compliance with such policies and expectations. For example, while one clinician may see all clients on time, another may routinely make them wait in the waiting room beyond the appointment time. While one crisis response nurse may drop everything when a client arrives in crisis, another may finish her lunch, gather up and read all previous documentation about the client, and then make her way to see the client an hour later. In such cases of variation, policy and monitoring of compliance (system issues) can standardize and improve these parts of the client experience by not leaving such important matters to the individual discretion of staff members. However, that is still only helping to improve the individual level of client-centeredness.

Client-centeredness is more than just those interpersonal interactions between staff and clients. It is also an issue of process design, procedure development, policy construction, approaches to troubleshooting crises, approaches to handling complaints, actual methods and criteria for making management decisions, and so on.. These are the critical elements – the *stuff* that connects together all the work of the individual pieces (staff).

It is the glue. It is the collection of bridges between services. It is the methods and the paperwork that allow a client to get into and out of the program. It is the forms and the steps taken to allow two clinicians to help the same client when needed. It is the physical structure of the waiting room. It is the decision about what part of the program gets more or less money. It is the scheduling of staff meetings, the recording and sharing of client information, and the days and hours of operation.

Leaders and managers in these public programs engage in decisions and actions in relation to these things on a daily basis. All of these kinds of issues combined make up the system. That is what needs to be reconceptualised and changed, not necessarily the clinicians, nurses, admin support, or any other staff members. They are doing their jobs, caring for clients, and doing so according to the established or normal processes. If those processes themselves are driven by priorities other than the clients' best interests, then the work staff do, while caring for and caring about a particular client, may not actually end up being what is best for him. That is not the fault of the staff person. That is the result of a *system* not being client-centered. It is the result of longstanding processes designed to meet needs related to data, money, control, bureaucracy, efficiency, or professional biases.

While most staff hired into such programs are compassionate either by nature or nurture, and have become client-centered practitioners through formal education and training, the systems they come into when hired have rarely been designed to be truly client-centered. This book is intended to help move us into that kind of intentional reforming of the system, within a client-centered paradigm built for that sole purpose. In achieving that, all parts (staff), procedures, spaces, paperwork, policies, and common practices will comprehensively, predictably, and reliably conspire to create a positive client-centered experience for those needing help.

Beauty Client-Centeredness is in the Eyes of the Client Beholder

Listen to clients, spokespeople, or advocates who come to us through the media. Listen to those who file complaints directly with mental health and addiction programs. You will hear many specific details about individual cases that on the surface appear to be diverse and unrelated. One person might be frustrated by waiting too long for a first appointment, or even getting the first one but waiting too long for the second or subsequent sessions. A client may be annoyed and confused about needing to see one therapist for his depression and another for his substance use, and may even lose much needed income by having to attend more appointments than would seem necessary. Another may experience exacerbation of her anxiety by having shown up on time or early for her appointment, only to find herself still in the waiting room 10, 20, or 30 minutes after the scheduled appointment time. Yet another may be offended by the fact that he is being asked questions someone else in the same program has already asked on a previous occasion. Or, perhaps someone feels their issues are being either dismissed or over-medicalized.

The list goes on, and perhaps many readers could write pages and pages on their own experiences with the system. Regardless of the specific circumstances, virtually all client and community dissatisfaction is based on a single theme – the perception that the system is designed to function in a way that puts its own needs before the needs of the client. To paraphrase the all too common client and public perspective, *it's not about us.*

Clients want to see and feel that the attitudes, decisions, actions, and processes they experience are based primarily on their needs as *the* priority over the needs of the system. Those of us who have been part of running these programs can easily come to believe that our systems and procedures are justified for all kinds of reasons (e.g., money, efficiency, our need/desire for data, staff convenience or preference, avoidance of union grievances, protecting our turf/mandate). Such rationalizations can allow administrators to feel comfortable making system-centric decisions, and remain unaware of the wrong-mindedness of this approach. It may even allow some to believe their systems are client-centered, and to not really notice evidence to the contrary coming from all the clients who are negatively affected.

Mental health and addiction programs need to function, to the greatest extent possible, in a client-centered fashion. The essence of the concept lies in a simple question. If your sister, brother, son, daughter, mother, father, or partner were the client, how would you want or need the program to function, aside from having compassionate people working there? If you are working in the system, this is an absolutely-critical question to ask at every decision-point in the redesign or transformation process. Imagining the client is a loved one is essential.

If we imagined *ourselves* as the client, instead, it would not have the same impact because we could choose to demonstrate patience and acceptance of flaws (rationalization again), and thereby not be bothered by some of the system-centric features of our programs. We tend to have less tolerance for our loved ones being ignored, dismissed, disrespected, or their needs being insufficiently or inappropriately addressed. Client-centeredness of a system depends on empathy in those designing it, not just those providing the care. Leaders must be able to imagine what the experience of a client would be under various policies, processes, and structures. They must be able to envision and relate to how a client would experience all decisions affecting provision of client services.

As a leader/manager, imagine it is your family member and how s/he would experience your decision or approach. An administrator might think the services are client-centered, until asking this simple question. Suddenly, with that change in perspective, the picture is different Client-centeredness is in the eyes of the client.

Actions for system managers and leaders:

Base every decision on what you would want for your loved one if s/he was the client, and on what you would believe to be the best experience for him/her. Use empathy, not rationality. Ask clients and their supporters for advice on system design, then use it.

Actions for clients, supporters, and advocates:

Regularly provide information directly to the program managers, leaders, and politicians about your experience with the mental health and addiction programs, so they understand how different parts of the system feel from the client perspective. They need to know both the good and the bad. I am not suggesting just tearing it apart. I am suggesting that you help them understand what it is like.

Wait Times from a Client-Centered Perspective

Even the way we track and report data regarding wait times can be consistent with either a client-centered approach or a system-centered model. Across health care, we have many kinds and versions of client data systems that help track wait times, length and frequency of service, and so on.. Of course, the Achilles heel of these systems is that they suffer from what a brilliant and hilarious computer technology colleague of mine calls a biological interface problem. They rely on the validity and reliability of the data being entered in the system. These are affected by consistency of training, interpretation of the data fields, and accuracy of data entry among all those creating or entering the data. What does it give us in the end? Even if it is reasonably accurate data going in, it still only represents a system perspective of what wait times are. Such data is not derived or presented from a client-centered view.

Imagine the client is your brother. What would you want to know? What form of wait-time question would really be relevant and useful for you and him? You would likely care very little about what the data system says is the average wait time of the service over a certain period of months or years. That might be either encouraging or discouraging. The only question that really matters for you and your brother is when his appointment will actually take place, and how long he will have to wait for it. That is what wait time really means to the client. For instance, at the time of writing this book, the posted wait time for the south shore of Nova Scotia for child and adolescent mental health was 42 days (the lowest in the province). In reality, however, children are being seen within 21 days and adolescents in 1-7 days. So, if a person was looking for help, that is the real time he would wait... the real wait time.

This discrepancy presents a problem because people's expectations, based on the published information, can affect their engagement in services. For example, if you were to look at the posted times, and get the impression that your child/adolescent would be waiting almost two months to see someone, how would you respond? What would your feeling of discouragement as a parent lead you to do next? For many parents, one of two things might go through their minds. They might conclude this system to be of no use, and that there is hence no point trying to seek help. Alternatively, they might believe their child's problem to be more urgent and/or serious than that, and take her to the emergency department of a local hospital. The first of those responses is simply tragic. The second directly worsens our ongoing struggle to have the emergency department used only for emergencies, and to have other issues dealt with at a more appropriate spot in the continuum of care. All this despite the fact that quick access may have actually been available sooner than what the posted information indicates.

Let's look at the opposite example. Suppose your teenage daughter needs mental health care. You have heard lots of bad things about wait times, so you check. The posted times tell you that there is an *average* wait of only three weeks. You call to get an appointment, and discover that the date offered to you is six weeks away. This may be due to fluctuations in staff absences, retirements not yet replaced, and seasonal variations in the demand on the service. Nonetheless, the problem, and your reaction in this case, is obvious. This just contributes further to the longstanding mistrust of the mental health and addiction system. You may feel very discouraged and hang up frustrated and angry, or you may decide that is unacceptable and head for the emergency department, so we are back to the same problem.

From a client-centered perspective, there is only one wait time. There is only one way to measure it. If I call today, when would I get an appointment? It is not a static variable, and does not have stability or consistency over time. The true test, and the only one that we used as our measure while transforming our system in South Shore Health, was an immediate client-centered perspective. When we wanted to know how we were doing on wait times, we would simply talk to an intake worker, and ask the question "If I were a client and called you today with a regular, non-urgent need, when would my earliest appointment option be?" That is the measure that matters from a client-centered perspective. That needs to be the target of all our work. That is the only true indicator of the extent to which we are meeting the client's needs regarding wait times, as opposed to the system's need for data that rolls up into an overall average picture. That rolled-up average has value to the system, but not to the client.

One caution is that some programs have an initial step before a client *really* starts having a meaningful clinical conversation about his concerns. These may be intake interviews, screening or matching interviews, and so on. In any case, from a client perspective, they don't really count unless the client actually gets to start talking about, and getting help with, his own self-identified needs. Those other meetings are part of the administration and client placement/flow process of the system. Preliminary meetings that are mostly for information gathering (e.g., structured interviews, screening or assessment tools) or streaming of clients (e.g., matching meetings), are generally not experienced by the client as helpful to them. They are experienced as the system putting them through steps that meet its own efficiency needs. Therefore, if a client hasn't started actually being helped, then the client is still *waiting* to start being helped. So, throughout this book, when I talk about wait times, I am referring to the amount of time a client will actually wait to start a client-directed, supportive or clinical discussion about his needs and issues. In other words, how long will he wait before the start of his being helped?

> **Actions for system managers and leaders:**
>
> 1. Regularly (weekly or monthly) check the true wait time for a new client calling in, and use that both as your quality improvement indicator, and as the number you report to the public. Its reality-based nature from the client perspective will serve you well in your transformation processes, and clients will always be accurately informed.
>
> 2. Don't use screening or matching appointments as the indicator if the provision of meaningful help does not actually start at that appointment. If it was your mother, which appointment would you consider to be the beginning of her feeling she is being helped? Use the wait time to *that* appointment as your indicator. That is the one that is about the client, from the client's perspective.

> **Actions for clients, supporters, and advocates:**
>
> Check with your local programs to find out how long your family member would wait if she called today for an appointment. It is public information, not private, so you should not have a problem getting that answer. Then rely on that number, not whatever is published.

"Client", "Patient", or "Person"?

Virtually every health care organization, as well as most other kinds of social services, businesses, etc., uses some type of terminology that conveys the importance of the client, customer, or person it serves. In health care, specifically in the acute care field, one will hear, or read on a plaque on the wall, statements about being *patient-centered*. From people working in more community-based kinds of health care, one may hear claims of being *client-centered*. More recently, as health care organizations attempt to bridge the gap between acute care and community-based services, more-generic language has been sought. In such cases, one may now see this referred to as *people-centered* or *person-centered*. All these ways of expressing the concept have advantages and disadvantages. Because of our historical use of some of these terms, they have taken on connotations that can be limiting or misleading. The words we use can affect the way we make decisions and design systems.

The word patient, for instance, is generally understood to refer to a sick person who is receiving medical treatment. That tends to be true in an acute care setting but clearly does not apply to all community-based services that health systems provide. In mental health and addiction programs, many people seeking help do not require medical treatment. Furthermore, if we create services that truly meet the demands and needs of the population, a very high proportion of the services we provide would be for people not considered to have an illness or a disorder. They would instead be for the promotion and maintenance of health through preventative and early intervention activities with people who are not ill (these concepts are discussed at length in later chapters).

So, the use of the term patient-centered, while having a clear meaning to medical professionals in acute care settings, only refers to some of the population we serve. Furthermore, it may be argued that the use of this term could create conceptual barriers to our fully understanding and embracing our legitimate and necessary work on the earlier end of the health and illness continuum. Across the whole system, this includes public-policy-based health promotion and targeted prevention activities. Within mental health and addictions, this also includes early supportive services for people dealing with trauma, stresses, and struggles in life that only require support now but could require more-intensive treatment later if unaddressed. The term *patient-centered* has noteworthy limitations, therefore, because it only refers to a small proportion of those we need to be serving. It only refers to people who are ill and need medical treatment.

The term *person*-centered is a broad attempt to be inclusive, and not to get caught in debating semantics (e.g., patient, client, customer). While it does accomplish that goal, it also carries with it a fairly significant limitation. It fails to address the issue of priority. It is silent on the question of *which* "person", or category of "people", is actually at the *center*. In other words, it does not indicate *who* is the system's priority. The term "person-centered" is also meant, presumably, to allow for the fact that the people we serve are important, but that our staff, volunteers, and other health care providers are also important. By using this general term, all those people can be considered to be included. It leads us to recognize the value of employee health and well-being, respectful workplaces, and supportive environments.

Of course, staff health is necessary and is absolutely *one of* the priorities of any employer in any sector. However, we still find ourselves running head-on into complicated decisions that have *competing* priorities. In such cases, we need to be clear about which competing interest comes *prior to* the other. It seems reasonable to argue that, other than in specific situations that constitute unavoidable exceptions (such as risks to staff safety), the person we serve must come before the people doing the serving. Sounds simple, and it is assumed most readers would agree in principle.

There are also times when financial limitations are firm and absolute, and implicitly construct limits around what can or can not be done. In such cases, those financial restrictions often take their place as *the* priority (e.g., budget cuts, service reductions, inability to expand to meet growing needs). However, regardless of deficits, if someone shows up in an emergency department in cardiac distress or displaying clear risk of harm to self or others, nobody questions whether or not we have the money to call in a cardiologist or a psychiatrist. That is because, in such life and death incidents, we seem to have our prioritization in order, such that our systems are centered around the immediate life-sustaining needs of that person.

Some of these kinds of acute-crisis situations, while they may have variability, are reasonably black and white and absolute in nature, and we tend to have a high level of consistency in our adherence to appropriate prioritization. But, what about the more-common systems and processes the majority of our clients experience every day in situations that are not life-or-death emergencies?

Imagine that a clinician is working on client case notes, and his next client arrives on time for an appointment. Should he drop what he is doing to see the client immediately, or finish his notes and then see the client 10 minutes later? The notes are important, but how does that compare, in priority, to seeing the next client?

Imagine that staff do not want to work evening hours seeing clients because that would be personally inconvenient for them. Should the organization schedule evening appointments to meet the clients' needs, or meet the staff request for only daytime hours, and maintain their work/life balance and their satisfaction at work? These situations occur daily, in which the needs or best interests of one *person* (the employee) compete with those of another *person* (the client).

The term *person-centered* fails to provide guidance or direction, and remains ambiguous, allowing for individual interpretation. Our programs and organizations do not exist for the primary purpose of meeting the needs of staff. Programs are not funded to ensure convenient work for managers or clinicians. They do not have a mandate from government or the taxpayer to make sure staff are scheduled to work *only* Monday to Friday daytime hours. Public health services exist for one purpose only. They are funded to meet the health needs of the public. Their job is singular, and in no way is it intended to be watered down or diminished by other important competing pressures.

I am not at all saying that we should ignore the well-being of staff or management. We have both a moral and legal obligation to ensure a healthy workplace, and, if we want to retain staff, we also have a pragmatic obligation to engage staff in meaningful and sustainable work. But, that is still not our actual purpose. For those of us who have worked in such programs, we must remember that our purpose is to meet the needs of clients, and, while doing so, must take care of our staff and volunteers. The former is the purpose, and the latter is part of the context in which we do that work. The former is the priority, and the latter is one of the other important things we must continue to address while doing our priority work. The bottom line is that *it's not about us (staff)*, it's about the client.

For these reasons, the term *client-centered* is used in this book as the descriptor of this suggested paradigm. Patient-centered implies only medical intervention for illness and disease, and keeps us from recognizing our important non-acute, community-based, health-oriented (as opposed to illness-oriented) work. People-centered is too vague and does not tell the leaders and the staff in the system *which* people come first, or *which* people are at the center. Finally, as discussed in a later chapter, the word *client* can refer to a community or a population, which further argues against the use of the terms patient-centered or person-centered, as they do not allow for the plurality of an essential population-focused approach.

The word client merely identifies the recipient of a service or a benefit from an organization. It is neither too precise and limiting nor too broad and vague to guide prioritization day to day. The term client-centered connotes, explicitly and unambiguously, that the needs of the client (whether an individual or a population) come before the needs of the system or the other people who work in it. It says that the people being served (the clients) are more important than the people doing the serving (staff, management, health care providers). This clarity and guidance is essential. Words matter.

Further Clarification of Terminology

The word *services* is used in this book to refer to the specific components of help, support, and treatment provided to clients, and so may include reception, counselling, therapy, and so on.. The word *program* is used to refer to the set of services which exist together in an organizational and operational structure in any geographic area. The word *system* is described at length above, and is used in the book to refer to the normative set of client and administrative processes and structures, and the usual and predictable types of interactions between people and organizations, that make up the programs and services we call mental health and addictions. The words *paradigm* and *model* are used to refer to the dominant beliefs, assumptions, perspectives, biases, and even culture that determine how we conceptualize and structure the mental health and addiction field and the people and programs within it.

CHAPTER 2

THE CURRENT TRADITIONAL MODEL; IS IT NECESSARY AND SUFFICIENT?

Traditional Approach in the Mental Health System

If we look at the dominant historical paradigm for these services, we find some interesting and problematic things. In the previously-separate mental health system (before any integration with addictions), we find a dominant pathology-oriented paradigm. This is essentially a psychiatric/medical model focussed on assessment and diagnosis of conditions that meet the criteria for psychiatric disorders in accordance with the Diagnostic and Statistical Manual (DSM). That means it is designed to look for and treat the most serious mental illnesses. This is not really surprising. The most dominant professions in the field have historically been psychiatry and clinical psychology, both of which are trained specifically and almost exclusively to identify, assess, diagnose, and treat psychological and psychiatric disorders. The guide book for all of that work is the DSM. It is based on ongoing empirical and clinical research, and translates that into a process for making a diagnosis. It provides lists and clusters of symptoms, and specific criteria to look for in a client, to determine if he may be diagnosed as having a certain disorder.

It is also exceptionally common for leaders and managers in mental health services to have worked extensively as clinicians in the system before taking over a leadership role. Most often, they are clinical psychologists or clinical social workers. This means they typically come into leadership roles having learned the system within its pathology-oriented paradigm.

The leadership and the culture of these programs have always been heavily influenced by psychiatry, as well. In the past, that may have been informal or unstated but it happened, nonetheless, because of the tradition-based perception of the power and expertise of physicians in the health system. In more recent years, it has been formalized as a head/chief of psychiatry, or a clinical leader kind of role. Currently, there is a further move toward formalizing a co-leadership model in many areas between a director/manager and a psychiatry lead. This is meant to be a way of bridging the gap between administration and medicine, and of ensuring greater engagement of physicians in the running of the system. Putting aside, for now, thoughts as to whether or not this is good, the one certain thing is that it will further support the traditional pathology-oriented paradigm on which the system is currently built. Decisions will be made jointly by a psychiatrist and an administrator who is typically a clinician.

What might we expect to see as the consequences of having had that pathology-oriented model dominate the evolution of the mental health field? First, we might be aware that, no matter what paradigm guides the development of a service, there will be side effects and unintended results. That does not mean the original intentions are wrong or the planned features of the system are not necessary. This is no different than taking any type of medication. There are intended effects – those we do need and which we use the medication to achieve. At the same time, there are side effects and unintended symptoms. The task for each of us in such a case is to weigh out the advantages and disadvantages of that medication. If the advantages of the intended effects are worth the disadvantages of the unintended consequences, then we continue to take the medication.

Now, let's take a look at the two sides of this equation for the mental health system. The same complication exists in these kinds of public services. A service may be based on a need to do one particular thing. It might do it very well (like the intended or main effect of a medication), but still might fail to address other issues, or could even cause harm (like the side effects of a medication sometimes do).

The traditional, pathology-oriented medical model has allowed us to develop the ability to diagnose and effectively treat some psychological disorders. That is the strength of the model. That is the strength of the DSM, the clinical research, and the ongoing development of clinical and pharmaceutical interventions. However, it is important to understand that all health services are designed around *inclusion* criteria, such as the DSM diagnostic categories.

Inclusion criteria is a term used to describe the symptoms or charac-teristics that a person *must* have in order to be *included* in the service. For example, if you go to a flower shop, you will quickly discover that they will not sell you a bed. That is because you do not meet their inclu-sion criterion. In order to be their customer, you must be someone who wants to buy flowers. That is their inclusion criterion. Diabetes clinics are designed for a target population, those diagnosed with diabetes. Cardiovascular clinics are designed for those diagnosed with heart con-ditions. Emergency departments are designed for people experiencing a medical emergency. These are all general examples of inclusion criteria.

One interesting and important thing about inclusion criteria is that the application of them implicitly causes *exclusion*. One cannot exist without the other being caused. You can't define whom you *will* serve, without that automatically meaning that all the other people are the ones you will *not* serve. The minute you draw the line to determine who *can* be a client, you are clearly stating who *cannot* be a client. These two are completely interdependent and inseparable, like two sides of the same coin. Inclusion and exclusion are relative terms by nature. That means they only exist in relation to each other, and each one completely depends on, and reflects the mirror image of, the other.

This inclusion/exclusion issue has had practical implications for mental health programs. By saying (implicitly or explicitly) that we treat people with psychological and psychiatric disorders as our primary mandate, we automatically exclude anyone not meeting such criteria. A person who is having mental health problems of a more minor nature, which don't meet the diagnostic criteria of DSM, doesn't qualify. This is certainly part of the perception often held by the public. People have commonly seen the program as being hard to get into, and not just in terms of wait times. They have perceived the need to *qualify* by having a serious-enough problem. They have felt the system is *not about them*, the people who need less-intensive help. They have felt the need to try to convince someone that their problems are actually serious enough to justify help.

This is one of the reasons it is not uncommon that other health care providers exaggerate the symptoms in referrals to mental health services. Some have even engaged in a regular practice of indicating possible suicide risk when making a referral, even if there is no real evidence of anything imminent. Such a designation helps to ensure the client is perceived as meeting the inclusion criteria, and also helps to raise the triage level (level of urgency) and, thereby, circumvent the unacceptable wait times.

I have heard the mental health program commonly referred to as a **castle** with a moat around it. That was the metaphor used more often than any by members of the public and other health care providers. The tragic part is that all the good, caring people and skilled health care professionals working within the program were not to blame. It is not the fault of the psychiatrists, clinical psychologists, social workers, counsellors, therapists, managers, admin support, or anyone else. They were all doing their good work within the established paradigm, which itself was the problem. Compassionate health care was being provided, but within a castle (the system) that most people couldn't access unless they were the most-seriously ill.

I am not necessarily saying this traditional framework of pathology-orientation was ineffective, but does it help us move forward and improve the system? Is it needed in order to ensure the health of the public? Is it enough, or is it missing some components or features?

Is the Traditional Paradigm Necessary *and* Sufficient?

One way to look at whether or not a program is working well is by examining both the necessity and sufficiency of what it does. Simply put, if a program approach or model is necessary, that means it is *required* in order to address some or all of the needs of the people being served. It means it is needed and the people being served could not do without that program or that approach.

In the terminology of this book, a program would be client-centered if those who are served receive what is necessary for their care. Sufficiency, on the other hand, is a completely different issue. The question here is whether or not a program or system is *enough* to meet *all* the client needs. Does it adequately (or sufficiently) meet all the needs of the population the program is intended to serve? So, a program is providing client-centered service if it has a *sufficient* array of services, in the right quantities, to meet the diverse individual needs of each and every person it is intended to serve.

It is reasonable to assume that the work done by the mental health system, within the traditional, medical/psychiatric paradigm, is necessary. There are many people experiencing diagnosable pathologies that require medical and/or psychotherapeutic assessment and intervention. For people with such needs, there is no alternative. There is no acceptably-effective substitute. Therefore, necessity is covered. This traditional model of using DSM-based diagnoses and psychiatric or psychotherapeutic treatment is unquestionably necessary. Now… is it sufficient?

In order to answer this question, we have to look at the nature and total scope of the needs of the population. If we think of mental health and illness as a continuum, from optimal health to severe illness, it is easier to consider what is needed. There have been many iterations of this kind of graphic in health care. Seeing it in this form helps us understand the whole picture better, rather than each of us seeing only the one part of the continuum we may be most familiar with in our own personal experiences and observations. This illustration is not meant to be as rigorous an examination as some more formal models are. It is merely used to help us think about how our levels of health flow from one extreme to another.

healthy	at risk	early symptoms	moderate illness	severe/persistent illness

At the far right of the continuum, we have people with conditions for which a traditional pathology-oriented system is appropriate. They are experiencing illness that is identifiably severe, persistent/chronic, and is significantly disrupting their lives. These conditions often require medical/psychiatric treatment, and, in many cases, are best addressed or at least initiated in a specialty hospital setting.

Now, let's move a little bit to the left on the continuum. Here, we might find people who are experiencing troubling symptoms of mental illness that are disrupting their lives, causing difficulties in their relationships, employment, for example.. While some may meet the criteria for a DSM diagnosis, and have symptoms severe enough to get across the moat and into the castle, some would not. Additionally, some clients would get in but be made to wait long periods of time because of being seen as less urgent and less than a perfect fit with the primary illness-treatment mandate of the program. Therefore, this group's needs may be partially met by the traditional medical model, but not entirely.

This type of situation is one that I have heard of many times from primary care physicians. The doctor knows there is a problem, but still finds herself frustrated by what she experiences as a lack of responsiveness by the mental health program. She sends in a referral describing the symptoms and making a case that the client needs to be seen. Then, many weeks later, discovers that the client is still waiting, and that his symptoms and many areas of his life have worsened. Ironically, I have heard some relief in physicians' comments and tone in such situations (in addition to the anger and fear) because it then gives them a more severe case to try to *sell* again to the mental health system. In other words, the fact that a client's condition has worsened actually helps that person get into the *castle.*

In this area along the continuum, there are people who are really struggling with identifiable illness, but who are not the most severe or most urgent. So... they wait. Access is not equitable. Their level of access is lower than those to their right on the continuum. How does this compare with other parts of our health care system?

Well, we are certainly experienced with triage. Our emergency departments do this minute by minute of every day and night. They triage based primarily on immediacy and severity of risk at any given time. However, we must remember that technically speaking their job is *only* to address emergencies. Given how many people come in without emergent problems, strict triaging is absolutely essential in order to ensure such urgency does not get lost among the sore throats and general malaise.

Our mental health system, however, is not mandated with a scope that is limited to only the most serious or urgent. Its job is to address the mental health issues of all citizens seeking help. In the mental health system, everything from mild anxiety to severe psychosis or depression with suicide risk is part of the job. Unfortunately, the traditional mental-illness model has not always served people with less-serious problems because they don't meet the unstated inclusion criteria.

Looking further to the left on this continuum, we will find many people who are experiencing some mild to moderate symptoms of psychosocial or emotional difficulties. This might include, for instance, a person who struggles with higher levels of anxiety than other people when stressful situations arise. It may be a person whose level of affect (i.e., mood) is frequently lower than many of his friends. He is just less happy than most and can't figure out why or what to do about it. These are people who may require much-less-intensive help, perhaps in the form of skill building (e.g., coping skills, emotional intelligence coaching, relationship management skill development). These are not people who necessarily require a psychiatrist, a clinical psychologist, or any other type of profession or service that focuses on the diagnosis and treatment of disorders. In many cases, such people could require more of a counselling and skills-training service, which historically would not have fit with the mandate of the traditional mental health system. This is another example of people in need of help who are excluded from services by virtue of not meeting the stated or unstated *inclusion* criteria.

Proceeding further to the left on the continuum, we find people who are generally healthy but experiencing occasional difficulties, or living with various risk factors for mental illness. This may be someone who has experienced trauma and has not had help dealing with it, or is facing a very stressful event or period of time in her life, such as illness of a child, failing a course in school, being in conflict with a friend, or losing a job. It could be someone living in conditions of emotional or physical abuse at home, school, work, or even online. It might be an adolescent who has developed an addiction to cannabis, thereby increasing his risk of schizophrenia. Perhaps it is someone living in poverty who has no source of social support to help manage the incredible stress of such a life, or a person going through a divorce, or experiencing the loss of a loved one. These are all people who regularly or occasionally need some help managing challenges that will cause more-significant psychological problems if unaddressed.

What these people usually need is good-quality social support and guidance to help develop or maintain resilience, self-esteem, and coping skills, for example. Many people (but not all) have access to good *informal* social support. This is a term generally used to mean support from friends and family. Those who do not have that will require *formal* support, which refers to people in organizations whose job is to provide such help. Sometimes, this formal support is needed simply because the nature of the issue being dealt with is beyond the ability of the informal supporters, or because the person usually providing that informal support is the one that the individual is in conflict with or has lost. In any case, formal support is needed by many people in order to prevent exacerbation of the psychological difficulties caused by challenging times in their lives.

Our traditional psychiatric model generally has not recognized this work as being within its mandate. These more-minor issues don't even come close to meeting the inclusion criteria to receive psychotherapy or a psychiatric intervention. In one way, that is good because psychotherapy and psychiatry are not what these people need. But, the other options and services are not there. They don't exist because that work was never envisioned as part of the pathology-oriented program, by the pathology-oriented professions that built the system. The result is that our programs, while dominated by such a model, have left this entire segment of the population out. These are people who do not meet the inclusion criteria, so they are excluded. Tragically, our system's failure to help them when their needs are less serious will catch up on us because many of them will become more ill and eventually meet the inclusion criteria.

At the far left of the continuum, we find healthy people. These are people who are not experiencing symptoms of pathology, are not necessarily living with risk factors for mental illness, and do not necessarily require any kind of individual service or intervention. However, given that many of our more-severe and chronic types of illnesses (mental and physical) are caused and/or influenced by economic, social, and physical environments, this population presents an opportunity. Our system needs to be working to keep healthy people healthy.

While some of this work has been built into the staffing and budgets for addiction programs for decades, such population-focussed health promotion work was historically not part of the traditional model for mental health services. Therefore, the dominant model of almost exclusively treating acute illness has failed to contribute to meeting the health-sustaining needs of the public to be served. This concept is discussed in greater detail in a later chapter.

Taking this continuum into consideration makes one point very clear. Our mental health system's overriding focus on treatment of acute mental illness – within a pathology-oriented medical and psychiatric paradigm – is simply not sufficient. In theory, it is able to meet the acute needs at the far-right end of the continuum. The type of training received by psychiatrists, clinical psychologists, psychiatric nurses, and some others in the system is well suited for this acute care work. It is, therefore, a necessary component of a service for those with the more-serious illnesses. However, as the dominant paradigm, it seriously fails to help the larger number of other people needing a different kind of prevention, support, or early intervention. This is why a client-centered paradigm is what is needed as the dominant framework for the system.

Thinking about this issue in the context of a continuum, as we have been, is useful but limited. Many years of effort have been put into a more comprehensive approach delineated by Brian Rush at the Centre for Addiction & Mental Health (Rush, 2010). He has looked at this simple concept of a continuum and considered the distribution of people across all the levels. He then developed a more-sophisticated method for calculating and projecting the required amount and type of resources to address the various needs that exist at all points along such a continuum. The tiered model is often depicted in the graphic shown in Figure 1.

Figure 1 (on next page): Tiered Framework for mental health and addiction system and service planning (Rush, 2010)

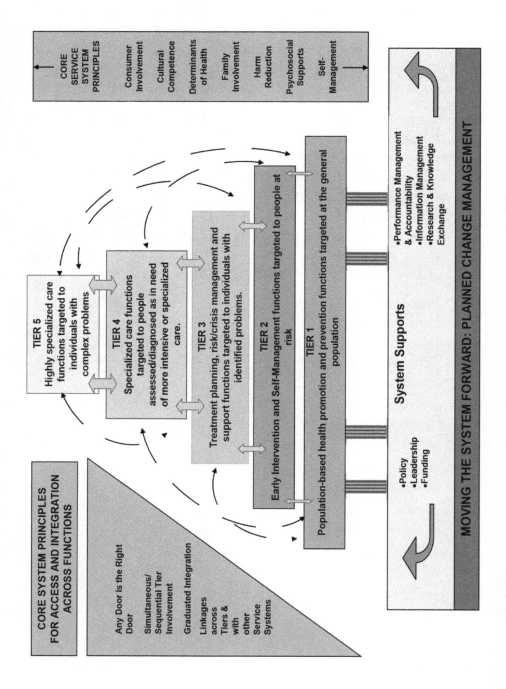

When placed in this format, we see very quickly that the most-intensive therapeutic interventions are only needed for a very small number of people at the peak of the pyramid. As we move down, there is an inverse relationship between severity of illness and number of people at that level. As we get near the base of the pyramid, it is obvious that a very large number of people are not ill but have a need for support, guidance, skill building, etc., in order to maintain their health. We also find an even-larger number of people at the bottom tier who are healthy, don't require formal supports, but do require a physical, social, and economic policy environment that will allow them to thrive and be healthy without interference.

Now, let's consider all of this in the context of the original question about whether our mental health services are both *necessary* and *sufficient*. We have already established that the psychiatric model of assessing, diagnosing, and treating people who are experiencing psychological disorders and serious disruption to their lives is necessary. However, it should be fairly obvious, when considering either the continuum or the tiered model, that the majority of people's needs are not met by such a service. If we are not providing robust supports and initiatives for the majority at the middle to lower levels of the tiered structure, then we are not meeting the mental *health* needs of the public we are mandated to serve. We are only meeting the mental *illness-treatment* needs of a select few. A program or organization cannot call itself client-centered if it fails to provide the kind of help needed by the *majority* of those people for whom it is responsible. It is easily argued that we don't have a mental health program, but rather only a *mental-illness-care* program.

It is reasonable, therefore, to conclude that our services, under that traditional paradigm of pathology-oriented psychiatric and psychother-apeutic program design and delivery, are *necessary* but *not sufficient*. It does part of the job well, but utterly fails at the health promotion, prevention, and early intervention components. Throughout this book, we will explore how a shift into a client-centered paradigm, and away from this more-limited psychiatric model, can correct this significant gap, while still maintaining those important traditional services for the appropriate purposes and clients. In other words, we need to take what is now an over-arching paradigm for the whole system, and move it into being simply one of several clusters of specialty services within a new and more inclusive paradigm called client-centeredness.

Traditional Approach in Addictions

Most of the previous discussion obviously refers to the mental health field since it has evolved as a separate and distinct entity from addiction services programs. Nevertheless, the addictions field has not been without its limitations.

Going back a decade or more, what we would find in the addiction field is a similar focus on the upper end of the continuum, but not based on the same diagnostic approach. As is widely known, much of the addiction treatment field evolved out of peer counselling being done by people who had experienced addiction and were in recovery. In the past, most of the people hired into the newly-developing, government-sponsored programs were those who had extensive experience with 12-step programs like Alcoholics Anonymous, and with an unwavering perception of addiction as a disease.

One of the key manifestations of addiction programs evolving out of disease-model-thinking is that it created inclusion/exclusion criteria at a functional level, based on client self-diagnosis. Someone having a problem with alcohol would come to an addiction program for help. Unless he was willing to talk about having an *addiction* and submit to the idea that abstinence was the only solution for the disease, he would be deemed to be someone who was "resistant" or "not ready for treatment".

The old-school, confrontational approach used in that conversation forced people to include themselves in, or exclude themselves from, that limited section at the far right of the continuum called addiction. For the longest time, the result was the same as described above in the mental health discussion. The system failed with a great number of people, in this case simply because they would not self-assess and self-label as fitting the criteria for that pathology. Over time, that began to change. The field began to recognize that it was able to help people reduce the harm that alcohol and other drugs were causing in their lives, even if that person was not necessarily an *addict*, or was not willing to admit to it.

I remember many years ago having taken over the management of a particular geographic area, with a collection of staff I had not met. I was travelling from town to town meeting each one, and trying to get to know them. In one small clinic, I arrived to meet with the only therapist based at that office. As I entered, he said, "You probably passed my client on your way in, as he stormed out. He was pretty angry." Okay, so if sparking my curiosity was the goal, mission accomplished. "Why was he angry?" I asked. I then almost immediately regretted asking because of the response I got. "Because I told him he was an alcoholic, and that he was not going to get anywhere in treatment until he admitted it. So he got mad and stormed out." I then indicated that I thought that was very unfortunate. The therapist replied, "No, I consider that to be a good clinical outcome." For readers who might be confused at this point, I will clarify that yes, indeed, he said it was a good clinical outcome, and that was not a typo on my part. I wasn't even sure what to say at that point, except I knew I had no choice but to look for an explanation, in hopes that there was something reasonable or rational in such a statement. So, I asked him to explain. "Because it proved that I was right and he does have an addiction, because I was pushing the right buttons," he replied.

As I have pondered that conversation over the years, a few simple truths continued to haunt me. First, and this one is pretty important I think... you can't counsel someone who is not there. So, if the therapist's approach caused the client to self-select *out* of treatment, then the therapist being "right" about the problem does not serve the client's best interests. It does, however, serve the therapist's ego, I suppose, except for the obvious flaw in his logic. If the client had an addiction, denial may cause him to storm out offended, as the therapist surmised. But, if the client did not have an addiction, and was being told he did (in that old-school, confrontational manner), what might his response be? Well, perhaps he might storm out offended. Either way, you can't counsel someone who isn't there. The second simple truth is that if our systems and approaches are attuned primarily to look for and treat problems at the most extreme end of the continuum, we will find them (whether they exist or not). We will also fail to help many more than we succeed with. Our somewhat forced self-inclusion criteria caused many to be excluded and unserved. There is an old adage that "If your only tool is a hammer, everything looks like a nail".

One of the main points to take from this history is that the addictions field itself relied heavily on client self-diagnosis for inclusion (*gently encouraged* through confrontation sometimes), rather than on assessment or diagnosis by a health care provider, or an expert. The advantage is that this approach is somewhat client-centered by nature (promoting a loose form of self-determination). The disadvantage is that it was likely responsible for our creating services that were less than efficient.

For example, our withdrawal management services (detox) have historically existed only as inpatient programs. It is only in more recent years that outpatient withdrawal management has been tried in Nova Scotia. Detox units may have had the loosest inclusion criteria of any health service ever created. If somebody self-identified the need to have a detox bed, she would almost always get the bed (as soon as there was one available). The person would call the unit to get on the list, and would be booked for admission at that time or during a later phone call. The client would show up, and go through an admission process, which included assessment of her addiction and medical issues.

If you have thought about the order of these events, you will have noted that there was no assessment to determine if this person met any particular kind of threshold or criteria to justify admission to an inpatient unit. Nowhere else in our health care system will you find this hotel-booking style of inpatient unit. People could be admitted because they needed a place to stay for a few days, and could use their mild-to-moderate substance use as the justification. People were admitted to detox beds for gambling addiction. In large part, this was merely a reflection of the political need to have treatment services appearing to offset the harm caused by government-sponsored gambling as a source of revenue generation. It was never precipitated by a medical need for a hospital admission.

On the question of necessity and sufficiency, this type of program was opposite to the mental health approach described earlier. This wide-open approach to detox beds was sufficient because it met everyone's needs and nobody was excluded. However, it was not necessary because for many people an inpatient admission and 24-hour medical supervision and treatment was simply not required. Appropriate treatment or support could have been provided in a less-intrusive way. That lack of necessity, and wide-open inclusion, caused serious wait time problems in some areas because beds were frequently full, and sometimes with people who could/should have been treated on an outpatient basis. As a result, people who actually needed beds had access problems.

Consequently, much of the work in this mental health and addiction field was necessary, but not sufficient, and other components were sufficient but not necessary. Programs were either under-treating or over-treating the population they were mandated to serve. The historically-dominant disease/medical model led to this imbalance. If replaced by a client-centered paradigm, these services would meet the needs of all those looking for help, but would do so in a way that properly fit each person's requirements.

Stigma and the Traditional Paradigm

There is a great deal of work being done to reduce stigma in mental health and addictions. Thanks to brave leaders and role models like Canadian Olympian Clara Hughes, we are taking on the challenge like never before. These efforts are essential for a variety of reasons. Stigma can cause people to feel marginalized from others, to feel like outcasts, to experience greater loneliness, depression, or anxiety. Stigma also causes people – because of many of these feelings – to stay silent about their challenges or their illness and to avoid asking for help. The issue we have not yet discussed publicly is that stigma can be caused or affected by the way we structure our programs and services.

The more we maintain the traditional dominance of the medical/psychiatric model, the more we sustain stigma. The more we adopt a true client-centered system and paradigm, the more we can potentially reduce such stigma.

Let's explore this further. The traditional approach described in this chapter for both mental health and addiction services, focused so much on the illness end of the continuum, contributes to stigma. It worsens the very problem we are now trying so hard to reduce. Stigma has its roots in social psychology and sociology. It is a form of stereotyping, which manifests itself in prejudice and discrimination.

A stereotype is a perception you have of people you consider to be similar to one another in some way. For example, we have a stereotype that people who wear glasses are smart, that Canadians are friendly, and so on. Stereotypes are fundamentally built upon our tendency to group or categorize people in our minds. We see certain people as having something in common with one another, and cluster them together as a group or as being the same 'type' of people in some way. When we draw a line around a group of people who we think are similar to one another, and determine them to be a certain kind of people, we are applying the same concept of inclusion criteria discussed earlier. We are saying that anyone with this particular characteristic is included in the group. By default, therefore, we are also defining exclusion. By perceiving some people to be in one category (tall), we implicitly are perceiving others to be excluded from that group and to be another 'type' (short). If you identify one kind of person as friendly, you may be implying that other kinds of people are unfriendly.

This connects further to the concept of ingroup/outgroup differentiation, from the very early days of social psychology. It is based on our perception that there are people like us and those who are not like us. In other words, the kinds of groupings we just discussed sometimes include us personally and sometimes not. When I think of a certain type of people as being similar to one another, and that group also includes me, that is what we call the 'ingroup', and by default everyone else is the 'outgroup'. If you identify yourself as being female, then perhaps you see women as your ingroup, and men as the outgroup. In that case, you might see women as 'us' and men as 'them'. We are constantly sorting the world in that way, between men and women, children and adults, Canadians and Americans. We are perpetually sorting people into **us** and **them**, based on thousands of different criteria. The more obvious the differences are between *us* and *them*, the more those differences will affect our perceptions of other people, and likely affect the way we treat them.

What I would argue is that the dominant pathology-oriented model described in this book has contributed significantly to stigma by causing the general public to see clients of either addiction or mental health programs as being different from them. Because of the psychiatric/medical/disease paradigm, this perception is actually valid and understandable. The fact is that the clients of these services have largely been **only** those with serious illness, especially in the mental health field. They have tended to be only people with diagnosable psychological or psychiatric conditions, or in some cases serious addictions. They have been mostly just the people with problems at the right end of the continuum or the top of the tiered system described earlier. They have not been people struggling and needing support with day-to-day challenges or risk factors in order to stay healthy. They have not been people experiencing early discomfort and minor symptoms that one day might become a psychological disorder if untreated. Instead, they have been that very small proportion of the population experiencing acute and/or chronic mental illness.

For the general public, it is easy, therefore, to follow the social tendency to discern differences between "us" and "them", and to see those with any kind of real illness as being *different… not the same… not like me… not one of us.* Therein lies the very foundation of stigma and the prejudice and discrimination arising from it.

We know that anyone going to a mental health program is mentally ill because we know *that* is *who* the system is designed for and who it actually allows in through application of the stated or unstated inclusion criteria. We know from many of our primary care physicians that anyone not ill-enough may struggle to get across the moat and into the castle. Therefore, it is understandable that the public would perceive and believe that anyone who *does* get in has a significant illness. By having a dominant paradigm in our system that is based on a psychiatric model, we have narrowed our actual client population to only those appropriate for such a model, and have excluded others. The clients in our programs, therefore, **are** different from the general population, but it has nothing to do with *them*. It is the fault of our system design, and we have placed them in the spotlight's glare so society can clearly identify them as different... and treat them differently as a result. Stigma.

If you imagine an alternative picture, one in which people dealing with all levels and types of minor and major difficulties in life were receiving help from mental health and addiction programs, how would that work? Well, people with significant psychiatric conditions would still be receiving service, which is essential. In addition, people with more-minor symptoms that have not yet progressed to being a diagnosable condition would be receiving service. People in need of support in dealing with stresses and challenges in life would also be receiving service. People simply needing to develop better skills in relationships, communication, coping with stress and trauma, etc., in order to stay healthy would be receiving service.

Now, think about all of this in the context of the pyramid or the continuum. We would have a service with which the majority of the population would feel comfortable, and that most individuals in the population would see as providing services that fit "people like me". Therefore, if I see it as a place that serves people like me, people who have my type or level of need, people who I might consider to be normal because they are similar to me, my perception completely changes. The idea of normal is one that really means I think they are like me, and I am like them. We each define it completely based on our own perceptions and our ingroup-outgroup clusters. Under this proposed new paradigm,

I would be unable to view clients of mental health and addictions as different from me. I would be unable to experience prejudice against people who need or receive help with these kinds of issues. That would be virtually impossible. We do not view people "like us" with prejudice or stigma, as we do with others we regard as different from us.

The bottom line is the more we can broaden the experience in mental health and addiction programs to significantly meet the diverse needs of a broader population, the less stigma will exist. The more we can provide services that are inclusive of the diverse levels of needs that people have, the less stigma there will be. One way to do that is to ensure that services are providing help to people all along the continuum, not only to those with more extreme conditions at the high end of the scale. We must provide service to more than just those who need psychiatric and psychotherapeutic interventions. We must serve the much larger number of people with lesser and more-common needs for support. This will also require a different approach to staffing, to be discussed later. Make a mental health service *normal* by designing it in such a way that everyone can see themselves in it, and receive help from it. A transition from a pathology-oriented paradigm to a client-centered paradigm would achieve this.

Actions for system managers and leaders:

Reduce stigma by maintaining psychiatric and psychotherapeutic services as **one** important piece of the program, but in addition develop non-psychiatric, non-pathology-oriented services for those healthy people who need support to maintain or regain their health.

Actions for clients, supporters, and advocates:

Advocate for the creation and expansion of early intervention support services for mild concerns and problems.

CHAPTER 3

CLIENT-CENTEREDNESS IN PUBLIC SERVICE VS. PRIVATE PRACTICE

Government-funded mental health and addiction programs often exhibit some characteristics of a private-practice model and have therefore lacked some of the features of what a public-service model should include. This is an important distinction because some of the private-practice characteristics I am referring to can inhibit a client-centered approach to service (if in the wrong context), and some of the public-service features that are missing can significantly enhance the client-centered nature of the service.

The term public sector refers to the array of programs and services that are paid for primarily by taxes (public dollars) through government. In Canada, this includes all health care – in theory. Of course, theory is not always the same as practice, so we still have huge amounts of the core health care system paid for through hospital foundations' and auxiliaries' fundraising, philanthropy, indirect user fees (e.g., parking), to name just a few. Nonetheless, let's leave that complex issue undebated at this point, and focus on the basic premise that our mental health and addiction programs, based within and/or primarily funded by government, are public services.

In addition, there is a large number of people delivering private services for mental health and addiction problems. In many jurisdictions they are primarily clinical psychologists, clinical social workers, and some forms of registered counselling therapists, because those are the main professions licensed to deliver psychotherapy. In addition, some psychiatrists work in private practice, but the bulk of their services are still paid for directly by public dollars, in which case it is not the same kind of pure private practice being described here. There are also various additional kinds of services for this client population being delivered in private practice by occupational therapists, recreation therapists, nurses, massage therapists, acupuncturists, and others. To be in private practice essentially means that the person delivering the client care services is paid by the client (or by his private health insurance policy) for the services, not by taxpayers. Even though the care providers may be compassionate and held to professional standards, it is a business model that, like any business, depends on being able to earn profit in the exchange between a customer and a company. This is not to suggest that this is necessarily a bad thing, but it is different from, and does not belong within, a public service.

In the next few sections, we will examine some of the important differences between these two models and some ways in which we have private-practice features in our public services. We will also consider the ways in which these two models contribute to, or detract from, our attempt to adopt a client-centered paradigm within our publicly-funded programs.

Transparency and Accountability

As a qualifier, I must state that people who go into any such health or therapy profession do so for the sake of helping clients to be well. Those in the private sector are no different from those working in a public health care service. They just work within a different system and paradigm. So, I am in no way questioning the integrity, intentions, honesty, client-centeredness, or skills of those in private practice. I am merely describing the systemic differences between the two sectors, and in particular describing the characteristics that a *public-sector* system should or should not include.

In a private-practice model, there is little formal requirement, if any, for transparency. The clinician, who is also often the manager or owner of the practice, does not need to demonstrate to anyone how she runs the business. There is no obligation to prove her time is being used efficiently because it is her own time, and it is her income that is negatively affected if not used efficiently. In such a model there is also no concrete way to ensure, for instance, that evidence-based approaches to therapy are being used, or that the systems/processes in that practice are designed for client convenience. Furthermore, even if there was a requirement for transparency and it showed the use of methods that had ambiguous evidence of effectiveness, or perhaps long wait times, the clinician is not formally accountable to any organization to change such things.

Simply put, despite the fact that most practitioners in private practice may be reasonably assumed to do good work with clients, there is little transparency or structural accountability in the private-practice model itself. To be clear, it may be argued that nobody has the right to expect such transparency and accountability in the operations of any privately-owned business. In any private business, this is actually appropriate and normal. But, do those same features and expectations belong in a public service?

The mental health and addiction programs in the public health care system are owned collectively by the taxpayers. Unlike the private sector, there is no profit mandate as there is no fee for the service. In a true public service, the level of transparency and accountability is or should be quite different from that in a private practice. In fact, it is expected to be and must be *much* higher. The more we subscribe to a client-centered system approach, the more important it is to build in such transparency and accountability.

As a program, our client is the public (i.e., the taxpayers). This is the population we are mandated to support, treat, serve, and satisfy. It is not limited to the individual level, or to those who choose to become a counselling or therapy client. Populations are our clients, and it is their overall health status we are mandated to improve. Those populations exist in many different forms and combinations. They are geographic populations such as the people of our province, city, town, or village.

We must also meet the distinct needs of the LGBTQ community, racial minorities, marginalized populations, geographically-isolated communities, those who have experienced trauma, and our ever-growing population of newcomers to Canada. Our client is the public, as a single collective, and it is to them that we are accountable through our elected officials.

We must be able to justify our decisions, actions, and expenditures of the money provided by the members of that public. We cannot make decisions that serve our own needs as individuals working in the system. We cannot make decisions that simply make our work more efficient, if it worsens the experience of the people to whom we are accountable. We cannot use public money to experiment with people's lives by using methods not demonstrated to be effective. One of my mentors once gave me and the rest of her leadership team a simple test to use with complicated decisions in a public-sector program – if a camera and microphone were put in front of you right now could you justify your decision to the public (the taxpayers who pay for the program)?

In private practice, there is no accountability of this specific kind. Accountability typically only exists in the sense that a registered health care provider is bound by a code of ethics and/or standards of practice that primarily prohibit the causing of harm. Accountability also exists on an individual level between the therapist and the client. Other than that, there is a great deal of freedom to practice according to whatever is agreed upon between the therapist and client. This is appropriate in the private sector. Again, I must state that my intention is not to criticize private practice, or the many skilled and compassionate clinicians who do that work, but merely to contrast the model with the public sector in relation to the features of a client-centered public service.

In publicly-funded programs, every decision, every minute, every dollar, and every person-hour of work time is owned by the funder and client... the public. We need to be able to demonstrate at any time that every bit of that resource is being used to improve the health of those people whom we are mandated to serve. The public has a legitimate right to know everything we do in a publicly-funded program, and to hold us accountable to do what is best for them. If every decision is not made with this absolute, formal accountability in mind, then our clients (the public – collectively and individually) are not at the center and are not the priority.

Language – My Clients, My Practice, My Office.

Language is capable of creating, sustaining, or changing culture. If we want to ensure a public-service kind of culture, we need to pay attention to language. The simplest way to convey and understand this is to say that there needs to be as much of a shift as possible from "I" to "we" across an entire program. Listen to the language used inside many traditional mental health and addiction programs. You will frequently hear terms like *my client*, *my practice*, *my calendar*, and *my office*. Sure, some of that terminology is needed to distinguish the work of one person from the work of another person. However, it is used not just in that discerning way, but, rather, as possessive or individualistic terminology.

Clinicians frequently become very protective of what they have come to consider their own practice, and their own clients. Many will reveal this whenever someone attempts to advise them how to handle a client, when to close a case, or why another clinician might be best for a certain client. Responses will include feeling offended, protective, defensive, and/or indignant that someone would presume to interfere with "my client" or "my practice".

This problem has been exacerbated by another bit of terminology regarding the relative roles of registered clinical professionals as opposed to paraprofessionals. In mental health services in Nova Scotia, people historically referred to paraprofessional staff (trained counsellors as opposed to registered/licensed professionals), or any staff with less than a master's degree, as not being qualified for "independent practice". Conversely, people who were said to be "master's prepared" were referred to as being capable of "independent practice". Part of the origin of the statement appears to reside with the profession of social work. Here is why.

In Nova Scotia, a master's degree in psychology has been the minimum requirement to become a registered psychologist, so there is no such thing as a psychologist with less than a master's degree. To become a registered counselling therapist (the newest psychotherapeutic designation in Nova Scotia), you must also have a master's degree. Nurses typically range from diploma to master's degree. However, it is rare to find a nurse in an outpatient, individual psychotherapy role because intensive training in such psychotherapeutic methods is not often a core component of nursing education. On the other hand, you can become a registered social worker with either a bachelor or a master's degree, but the master's is required if you plan to set up your own private practice. That is the distinction that leads people to use the term independent practice.

When people use this term, independent practice, they are sometimes referring to completing an assessment, formulating a diagnosis, and developing and delivering a treatment plan, without a more-qualified/ experienced or more-highly-certified professional endorsing or signing off on that work. However, the term has also been used to imply far more than that. It implies a level of freedom and disconnectedness from others. It implies the kind of autonomy that appropriately exists in a private practice. In other words, the therapist has the right to make all decisions about the way the practice itself functions, such as what kind of clinical work or methods will be used, or how many and which types of clients will be seen. That is essentially the nature of private practice. That same kind of private-practice language and implication has been sustained for many years in the public mental health system. In order to fix the system, this language must be changed to reflect a client-centered *public service*.

To change this, leaders in the system must spend a great deal of time and attention altering the language. They must repeat clearly and frequently key messages such as:

"This is not a private practice; it is a public service." and

"They are not **your** clients, or the clients of any one therapist, they are clients of the program or of the health authority... you are the health care provider assigned at this time to work with this particular person, who is one of the program's clients."

At all times, it must be made crystal clear that the *program* has an obligation to meet the client's needs, using whatever selection of services, staff, and approaches are most appropriate for that person's situation or condition. This may or may not continue to be any particular therapist if that is not what is best for the client. The therapists are not independent practitioners, as they would be in private practice, and so have no claim to the clients they serve. The clients are clients of the *program*.

Shared Space versus My Office

In our experience transforming the system, we also found it useful to designate all offices to be available for anyone's use when the primary occupant was not present. For instance, let's imagine there are 20 clinical staff, several clerical staff, and a manager working in a particular clinic. Imagine, as well, that staff from satellite offices sometimes come to work at this location for a few hours or days each week or two. Those visiting staff would likely work in a meeting room, or any available common area. This creates inefficiency, and does not really allow the visiting staff member to have a suitable place to see clients, or to have confidential client phone calls. This can be eliminated by making all offices available to such a visiting staff member, as long as it is empty at that time. This serves two purposes. First, it makes the most efficient use of all of the expensive office space being paid for by the taxpayer. An office does not sit empty if someone needs a space to work. Second, it reinforces the idea (by changing the language) that these are public offices, and no individual owns any of the space. That would be the case in a private practice, but should not be the case in a public service. In a public service, there is no individual ownership or claim to space. The employee does not pay rent for the office, the program does. And, while it makes sense for full-time staff in this line of work to have a primary workspace when possible, and to customize it for clinical comfort, sharing all such space among all staff who may need to use it is in the public interest (the interest of our client). That is what matters, not the interest of Joe the clinician or me the manager. *It's not about us*. It's about the client, and it's about the taxpayer who is paying us to make it about the client.

A Public-Service Schedule

The same principle regarding public service must also be applied to the issue of staff scheduling. Of course, we want staff to have some say in their schedule. This is important from an industrial/organizational psychology perspective. The more flexible a workplace can be in allowing people to manage the balance between their personal and professional lives, the more likely the organization is to have satisfied and healthy employees. However, while trying to provide that balance for staff, we must still start with the concept of the client being at the center. In other words, we must set out to create a staff/program schedule that would first provide flexibility and options for clients, but would also secondarily provide staff with an opportunity to have some control over the balance in their lives.

In many mental health and addiction programs, clinicians' schedules have historically been arranged almost entirely Monday-to-Friday, and during regular business hours. While there may have also been a few evening groups offered, if a client needed individual therapy, it would have to be scheduled during regular weekdays, regardless of whether he/she had to work during those times.

To make it worse, in many workplaces, a number of staff could be scheduled to work a 'modified work week' – a scheduling model in which an employee works slightly longer days each day, and then gets one day off every two or three weeks as a result of having worked additional time each day. Typically, the day of the week that staff would most often choose to have off was Friday. In practice, what that really meant was that almost all of the availability of appointments offered by the program ended up being between 8:30 and 4:30 Monday to Thursday. Furthermore, in some cases, the office would be closed for lunch (12:00-1:00) so that the clerical and reception staff could all be off for lunch at the same time.

Clearly, such scheduling does not reflect a system designed to meet the needs of clients as its top priority. This is not a way of functioning like a collective or unified service to the public. It is an example of a program functioning like a bunch of private practices, each setting its own schedule independent of the other's. To make scheduling client-centered, these are some examples of system variables that need to be changed to support provision of a true public-service model. The program would need to establish the overall hours needed by clients, and the staff would fit into that schedule, not the other way around.

In our experience within the former South Shore Health, we had many of these private-practice features in place as part of the traditional approach. We proceeded, therefore, to create a single (program) master schedule for all outpatient services. We advised clinicians they could propose their own schedules under certain conditions. For example, if any wanted to be able to have a day off every two or three weeks, or be able to come in late on a certain morning because it worked for their own childcare or family needs, etc., they could. However, they could only do so by working some evening hours offering appointments, and staggering lunches to see clients during the common lunch hour (to meet the clients' needs). We were prepared to assign people to evening hours, but we were looking for a win-win in how we went about doing it, by allowing staff to also make it work for their personal lives... as long as the client needs were met first.

This approach went a long way to convey the idea that we were not a collection of private practices. We were a single program striving to provide accessible services to clients, using a single, client-centered schedule, and using whatever staff and resources were most appropriate for the client need.

As we implemented this approach, it was fascinating to see the diversity in the reactions of staff. There were those who saw such an approach as a win-win situation, and voluntarily stepped up to help expand the clinic hours for the client. There were those who simply saw this as the right thing to do for the clients. There were also those who preferred to not take on evening hours, but believed in this direction and were willing to do so if asked. But, still, there were the few who could not envision the change or adopt the principle of making these decisions entirely based on what is best for the client. Those same few struggled to accept the rightness of making these decisions based on the program being a single, client-centered public service.

I recall one therapist specifically saying in a meeting that "We can try this evening hour thing but clients are not going to want those appointments". The evidence the therapist provided was that nobody had ever asked for evening appointments in the past. I found that to be fascinating logic because it implied that people would ask for something that they know is not available. We don't ask Walmart if we can buy a car from them because we know they don't offer that product. It is more reasonable to see this from the perspective of the often-quoted 1989 movie Field of Dreams – "If you build it they will come". In any population, we are going to find a diversity of scheduling needs. If, as a public service, we are going to try to meet the needs of that diverse public (our client), we need to offer a diversity of scheduling options. For the record, and not at all surprisingly, in our case those evening appointments were filled consistently once they were made available.

The small pockets of resistance and/or pessimism that can be seen during this kind of change, are just further indicators of people trying to hang on to private-practice thinking, in which they would each get to keep the schedule they preferred. Any of the arguments presented against this expansion of hours are additional examples of how we rationalize protecting the *status quo*. We rationalize keeping a system that is primarily designed to meet its own needs and the needs of management and staff, while avoiding the difficult and complicated change toward a client-centered paradigm. In any public service, a truly client-centered paradigm will not be achieved until the private-practice language and perception (e.g., my client, my schedule) are eliminated in favour of understanding that it is the health care organization that has clients, and it pays staff to help serve its clients.

Perhaps the greatest irony in this issue of scheduling is that, in reality, private practices are likely better at client-centered scheduling than the public sector. Working within a business model, a therapist must meet the scheduling needs of the client or suffer the consequence of losing that person as a customer (please forgive the corporate language – customer – but it helps make the point that a private practice clinician has a good reason to schedule around the client's availability). In a public service, staff do not make more or less money for seeing more or fewer people. Therefore, there is a disincentive in the system for catering to the scheduling needs of clients in order to get more clients in. It means more/harder work and no more pay. In private practice, client access and satisfaction directly affect the sustainability of the practice itself. This is yet another reason why we cannot allow the private-practice type of independence of each clinician within a public service. In that context, it is more likely to reduce access than increase it. These are very different models, and each is appropriate only when it is operating within its own sector (public or private).

Choosing Your Own Clients

In a private practice, a clinician gets to choose which clients he takes on. That is appropriate, given that it is his company, business, and practice. He can be selective about what kinds of psychological issues he will deal with, and can designate himself as specializing in a certain area. In a public service, this cannot be the case. The public health care system in Canada must take all clients indiscriminately. There is no kind of sorting and choosing that is appropriate in a public service other than triaging and appropriate case assignment. Our mental health and addiction programs must therefore function accordingly.

A common historical practice in this field is for a clinical team to meet and discuss new clients that have requested service (referred to as *intakes*). The client's symptoms and concerns would be highlighted, and any questions clinicians might have would be answered if the information is available from the intake interview. Then, there would be an opportunity for each clinician to choose if he/she was going to take on that client. While there was clearly an obligation for the *program* to provide service to each of those new clients, that responsibility was not translated to the individual-employee level. In practice, each clinician had the opportunity and the right to say yes or no to taking on any particular incoming client. As a result, the diversity of responses in these meetings was immense.

There were those in a team who would be the first to offer to take new clients and others with the entirely opposite response. There would be staff members who would appear to be in a 'world championship staring contest' with the table, staying as still as possible so as to not be noticed. If confronted or asked directly to take the new client, responses would include things like "I can't possibly take another one, I am swamped.", "Well I can take her, but I won't be able to see her for months.", or "I can't because I am already seeing that person's neighbor's cousin's wife." Admittedly, that last one was an exaggeration, but there were often questionable reasons offered for not accepting clients.

The majority of people working in this field are committed, hard working, and focussed on what is best for the client. However, the dominant structure/system had allowed for such a high level of individual discretion that huge inequities could exist. Ultimately, it was in the hands of each individual clinician to decide if the public dollar would be spent efficiently for the sake of more and better service to the clients. No public system should ever allow such personal-preference discretion on the part of individual staff members, because it is not client-centered.

In a private practice, this high level of choice would not be out of line because a company can choose to take or decline as many clients/customers as it wishes. In a public service, the program is accountable to the public (its client) to ensure all resources are being used fully. It is the program's responsibility to assign *its* clients to the people it pays to provide the health care. In a client-centered public-service paradigm, the intake system must be designed to assign clients directly to clinicians, and to ensure equitable distribution and full booking among all staff. Fortunately, throughout Nova Scotia at least, this is becoming a more common practice.

Standard Number of Clients and Appointments per Day/Week

Over the years, there have been many discussions and debates about the size of caseloads. One clinician might be carrying 60 clients, while another only 25. This field has struggled with the question of whether or not caseload size can be standardized. The simple answer is 'no'. Clients are very different from one another. Some are dealing with extremely complex issues that require intensive and comprehensive treatment. Others are dealing with needs that have more-straightforward solutions. Some need to be seen for long periods of time, while others can be helped with a brief intervention. For these reasons, the number of clients on any clinician's caseload is somewhat irrelevant. However, there is still a need in a public-service model to ensure the efficient use of tax dollars, in the form of staff time, and to ensure some level of equity among the staff. This can be addressed in a much simpler way than size of caseload.

It is quite possible to standardize the minimum number of clinical sessions provided, or minimum number of clinical hours spent, by any and all clinicians during the course of a day, week, or month. In the past, it was not unheard of in a mental health or addiction program for one clinician to be seeing five, six, or even seven clients per day, while another only two. In a very direct way, standardizing this component at least guarantees that our collective client (the public) is getting what it is paying for (a minimum amount of clinical time from the people it is paying to do the clinical work). Again, given the previous assertion that, in a public-service model, the term client can be used accurately to refer to the population, this whole direction toward minimum standards for the use of staff time is a move in the direction of being more client-centered.

There is an example that pointed out clearly for me the non-client-centeredness of private-practice features when applied inappropriately within a public-service program. During our primary year of transformation, we were working through several simultaneous changes. One of them was the standardization of number of sessions per day/week that each clinician would provide. Allowing for 60 to 90 minutes per session, and counting for time to do client-related phone calls, notes, case conferences, etc., we set it at four per day or 20 per week. We also accounted for clinical time spent facilitating client groups. Reactions to all of this were quite diverse. Those who were already highly productive saw this as perfectly reasonable, while others thought it was tight. In terms of our accountability to our client (the public) keep in mind that this was set as a minimum not a target. We still had people exceeding this amount.

Around the same time, we were also getting all staff to keep their schedules electronically on Outlook. Up to that point, as per the private-practice type of model, people were using all different forms of paper and computer methods to manage their calendars, and nobody really knew what was in anyone else's schedules. As a public service, that may have been a normal part of a lengthy history, but clearly was not appropriate and did not support a client-centered approach. What was missing was the transparency and accountability described earlier. If asked by the media or by government if all of our resources were being used efficiently, I would not have been able to answer with any certainty at all. We had to change that, so putting everyone on Outlook allowed management (as the designated representatives of the public and government) to see all schedules.

I had been watching for some time as certain clinicians repeatedly worked to sell the idea that they were busy. They were the ones who would rarely accept new cases and would claim that there would be a long wait time if they had to do so. I remember the day that I could finally look into all staff calendars electronically. I recall opening one particular therapist's calendar and discovering that, despite the impression people had, this person had only six appointments booked during the current week, only four the following week, and only two the week after. Everything past that point was pretty much empty. This was during a period when wait times were five months for adolescents and eight months for adults.

Putting aside the obvious issues of personal integrity here, this situation was directly enabled by the organization having evolved more like a collection of private practices than like a public service. If that therapist had been in a private practice, s/he would have gone out of business, but, safe within the old model of this public service, s/he was able to pull it off. The collective accountability as a public organization did not always translate to all individual staff members feeling the same level of responsibility to the public as our client. For the vast majority of the staff, that ethical commitment to the clients, and that constant high level of integrity, was always there. But, for that one or two, it clearly was not.

While addressing individual performance was and always will be a crucial part of managing such situations, the real flaw lies in the system itself. Its very nature enabled this behaviour. It needed to be changed to a true public-service model, in which the organization ensured complete transparency, program-driven standard levels of productivity, and no place for the rare but real work-avoidant individuals to hide. It is a public service that exists for the clients not for the people working in the system. *It's not about us.*

The Permanent Client

In a private practice, a therapist is able to continue seeing a client for whatever frequency or duration he/she chooses (if the client wants it, of course). It doesn't matter if there is a continuing therapeutic need or not. In such a case, there is no waste of resources or inappropriate use of time. Quite simply, a private practitioner is providing a service that a client has chosen to access and pay for. (Again, please don't take

66

such comments as my disparaging private practitioners. I am not. I am merely contrasting the nature of the private-practice *model* to that of a public service.) In a private-practice model, whether client involvement takes the form of 10 hours per week for four clients for 10 years, or thousands of clients for short sessions over a short term, is irrelevant. Clinicians may each have their own preferences, or self-imposed limits, or clinical approaches, but the model itself allows for any such variation in accordance with the choices of both the client and the clinician.

To a lesser extent, this same freedom has existed as a norm within many of our public mental health and addiction programs. Historically, it has largely been a clinician's decision about how long and how often she keeps seeing any particular client. There have been many cases in which a client has been seen every one to four weeks for five to ten years. Some of those cases have appeared to have no identified goals, no identified clinical issue, or no record of any identified psychotherapeutic method being used. In some instances, it appears that the clinician's role in the case has been not as a therapist but, rather, as a life coach or even a friend.

Why is this a problem in a public service? The first and most important reason is that it increases wait times. It takes up many hours of potential appointments that could be used to see new or previous clients who *require* active therapeutic care. This is really about using the right resource for the right reason. If there are clients who are stable, doing well, and simply need some kind of light check-in for social support or life coaching on an ongoing basis, the program needs to find the right way for them to receive that. There are various ways to proceed. First and foremost, if the job of the program is to help people and make them better able to live a healthy and independent life, then every employee must take intentional steps to prevent dependence on the clinician or the program. Instead of cultivating dependence, they should be working with the client to develop good social support systems among his friends, family, neighbours, and coworkers. In lieu of that *informal* social support, they may have the ability to offer a drop-in group for that purpose, giving people a place to check-in and keep feeling connected. This would support the client but not have the direct side-effect of preventing other clients with more current or active needs from getting in for an appointment. While a private practice does not have an obligation to keep making room for the public to access its programs, a public service does because the entire public is its client.

It is common knowledge that some of these long-term, frequent clients present much less work, and involve much easier and more pleasant sessions (although clearly some are very complex as well). For many, the relationship has been established, the therapist knows the client, and the communication becomes more relaxed and effortless. This is partially because, for many such clients, their need for long-term ongoing sessions with a therapist is minimal or non-existent because their need for *active* therapy has passed or is now sporadic (on an *as-required* basis). They need maintenance/support instead of therapy, yet are seeing a therapist. We are over-serving those clients. This is a mismatch of resource to need, and directly affects wait times.

In a public service, every hour of a clinician's time used for something other than the priority use of that position is literally another hour added to the collective wait time for a new client. Every seven and a half of those hours is literally another day added. Keeping the previously discussed definition of *priority* clear, programs need to decide between each long-term, stable client for whom a therapist is providing life coaching or social support and the many clients waiting to get in.

We can't pretend this choice doesn't exist. It does, and denial won't resolve it. Think of it this way. You are in an office tower, and you push the elevator button. The elevator arrives and the door opens. Inside is a crowd of people filling it from wall to wall. What do you do? Nothing, that's what. You wait. Now imagine that the elevator moves on, and you continue waiting. It arrives back again, and when the door opens, it has the same people filling it to capacity. This time one gets off. But, that is not enough to allow the five people waiting with you to get on. Having the same people continue to ride the elevator up and down and not get off, blocks access to that service. In mental health and addictions, the same basic principle applies. In any case where there is limited capacity, new demand cannot be accommodated if the previous demand keeps using all the capacity. People can't use the IN door, unless people also use the OUT door.

If you owned the elevator, and people were directly paying you to use it, then it would not matter in any way how long people stayed in it. There is no obligation or mandate to ensure access for the others who may be waiting. When the taxpayer has paid for it, on the other hand, and it is meant to serve *everyone*, there is such a mandate. It is the *right* of every citizen to be able to access that service. It is, therefore, the obligation of the program to ensure constant monitoring, and discharge or alternative service, of long-term clients who really need some other kind or level of care or support. This frees up appointments. Others can then have easy access to the elevator because some people were identified as no longer needing to ride it.

Evidence-Based Methods

The concept of evidence-based practice is an interesting one because our interpretation of it is determined by our own individual definitions of *evidence*. There are those who would say that if an individual tries a certain treatment and then believes he feels better afterward, that is sufficient evidence to claim the treatment method to be effective. Others would say that in some such cases what is being experienced is a placebo effect. What that means is we sometimes feel better just because we expect something will help us feel better.

For instance, we know that headaches and other kinds of pains and symptoms can either be reduced or eliminated if we are given a medication or treatment by someone who makes us believe it is effective. The expectation itself can cause that, even if the treatment really has no physiological effect on the pain or its cause. That is why, for example, drug companies must do what is called a double-blind randomized controlled trial to determine if a new medication actually works. The people in the experiment never know if they are taking the real medication or one that actually does nothing, like a sugar pill — called a placebo (incidentally, it is called a *double*-blind study because the people handing out the medication also don't know who is getting which pills).

Some of the people who take the real drug and some of the people who are only taking the placebo will feel better after taking it, even though we know the placebo is actually not doing anything chemically or biologically for the person's condition. After we take away the amount of perceived improvement caused by a placebo effect (thinking they feel better but not because of the treatment... only because of expectation), then we are left with the amount of real effect caused by the treatment.

As the debate continues, still others would argue that even if a person feels better in the case of a mere placebo effect, then the treatment provided has been effective for that person and cannot be disregarded. They would say that, even if a method has been tested and known to not actually improve a certain illness, if a person is led to believe it works and then feels better because of that belief, then it is an appropriate method to use.

Our public health care system has primarily evolved from a model that looks for scientific evidence of effectiveness. It asserts that, if a treatment actually works, we should be able to observe it working when compared with people not receiving that treatment, and we should see it working in more than just an incidental or anecdotal way. In other words, if half a group of people with a certain illness receives the treatment, and the other half receives just a placebo, the people receiving the treatment should end up with their illness improved more than those who only had the placebo. If both groups end up the same, then clearly the treatment doesn't work. It doesn't cause more change in the symptoms of the illness than a sugar pill. If it is a medication to eliminate a rash that appeared on your skin, and after treatment your rash looks the same as those who had a placebo, the medication did not remove or even improve your rash. People will always choose to believe what they want, and some will accept scientific evidence while others will not. That is our reality.

Permit me another story. I had a brilliant student from Zimbabwe in a course I developed at Saint Mary's University on applied leadership of social change. The issue he began to work on, which will likely be a lifetime pursuit for him, was to lead culture change in his home country regarding the acceptance of science-based medicine. He was not advocating that it should replace traditional healing methods and practitioners. Instead, he was advocating that people accept it as an effective adjunct or back-up plan for traditional methods when they fail to actually change a person's symptoms or health status. His plan to lead this change includes becoming a physician. He knows that one of the challenges he faces is the placebo effect caused by belief systems. He also knows he is tired, even at his young age, of watching people die because of placing their lives in the hands of some of the traditional methods that are less effective than others. Unfortunately, belief and expectations do not cure disease by themselves.

This complicated issue is very relevant to the private-practice/public-service distinction, and to the ways of conceptualizing client-centered, as well as having noteworthy ethical considerations. There is an interaction here. The way our definition of *evidence-based practice* affects client-centeredness, depends on the setting (private/public). Let's consider what this means.

Start with the fact – based on all the codes of ethics in our various health care professions – that it is unethical to mislead a client about the risks, benefits, and the very nature of a health care service we provide. Our informed-consent obligations require us to be forthcoming before treatment, so people know what they can expect to gain and what risks they need to be willing to accept. In other words, all licensed or registered health care providers are obligated by regulation to share the truth with each client about the best and most valid research evidence available. They cannot present a particular treatment method, which has no evidence of effectiveness, as an option without telling that client about the inconclusive evidence or about the evidence that it doesn't work. Keep this point in mind.

In a private-practice setting, as already noted, there is a component that is an agreed-upon service provider/recipient transaction. The practitioner is selling a service. As an independent service provider, she is obligated to provide the same information noted above, as part of the informed consent process. But, let's assume she believes that a certain treatment has some potential benefit based on anecdotal information from individuals who have said it helped them. She is able to have this discussion, be forthcoming about the ambiguous or non-existent scientific evidence, share the anecdotal comments, and negotiate whether or not the client wishes to participate in that particular treatment option. If the client chooses to proceed, he is doing so with the full understanding of the risk that it may or may not be effective at actually changing his health status. The practitioner is then free to provide any such service that the client is interested in, and that the practitioner is competent in delivering. Providing that the practitioner is not misleading the client into believing that the approach is fully supported in the evidence, and provided that the method does not cause harm to the client and is not restricted or banned in some way, she is then free to deliver that therapeutic intervention. It would not be considered unethical because there is full disclosure of its limitations.

Think now in terms of a public service. What is the mandate? It is quite different from that of a private practice. The public health care system is not really mandated simply to *provide* services. It is mandated to improve the health status of the individuals and populations it serves, *through* the provision of services. These may sound the same but they are not.

The mandate is to improve health or cure illness. The method of meeting that mandate is to provide services that are effective at reducing or eliminating the symptoms or illness. It cannot meet its mandate, therefore, if it uses methods that don't actually work. This is not exactly the same as with a private practice. In a private practice, the provider has more discretion to be able to offer services based on the requests or preferences of the client, and has no obligation to stick with *only* methods supported by *scientific* research.

The public system is not a business, and its services are paid for collectively by the taxpayer, with an expectation that they will *improve health*. That does not necessarily mean the bar is higher, but the options that should be considered ethically appropriate in the public sector are more limited. Since the real job is to improve health outcomes, the obligation transferred to the system by the taxpayer through government is to use methods that are most likely to affect those health outcomes. There is no room for individual negotiation of desired *services*. If a client wants to engage in a type of treatment that the empirical evidence says does not work, it would be an inappropriate use of taxpayer dollars (via staff time) to provide that service knowing it will likely not make the person's illness better. This public mandate changes the ethical context of the decision, when comparing a private practice to a public service.

Please be clear in understanding this does not imply that either situation is right or wrong. It is merely pointing out that the ethical obligations in these two contexts are different. The definition of acceptable evidence has more latitude in a private practice than it does in a public service. The clinician can choose to provide any reasonable service that a fully-informed client wants to receive. Therefore, the definition of evidence-based also varies from one context to the other.

When a client comes to a public health care service, he expects to be provided with services that will help fix the problem being experienced. That expectation carries an assumption of *effectiveness*. A private practice can offer services based on more-diverse kinds of evidence and still be providing professional quality client-centered service. The clinician is still meeting the needs and preferences of her individual client. However, when we recognize that the overall client of a mental health and addiction program is the public, the population, the taxpayers, then client-centered service can only be achieved if we are providing the most effective methods available with the expenditure of their dollars. That is the only way such a public service can meet the mandate provided by its client. Client-centeredness in a public-service model requires an intentional use of methods supported by scientific evidence in order to meet the expectations of its broad public client, but also to remain accountable for the most effective use of the funding provided (as per the earlier discussion on transparency and accountability). It must work to achieve the mandate of improved health outcomes, using methods that will accomplish that.

> **Actions for system managers and leaders:**
>
> If a public mental health and addiction program under your responsibility is using methods that are refuted or unsupported in *scientific* evidence, after placebo effect is accounted for, terminate that service and reallocate the taxpayers' money toward methods that affect the mandated outcome of *improved health status.*

> **Actions for clients, supporters, and advocates:**
>
> If your local program is spending time and money using methods that you know are shown to be ineffective in this field, other than placebo effect (acupuncture has been one such commonly-used ineffective, but placebo-inducing method), advocate for that use of your tax dollars to be stopped so the program becomes more effective.

Two-tiered System

Psychotherapeutic services are one of the areas of Canadian health care in which we allow for a two-tiered system. That is, we allow there to be a publicly-funded system, but also allow for a parallel privately-funded system. Conceptually, this is more similar to American-style health care, which we know to be a less effective approach to looking after the health of its citizens. A key reason why it is a less effective model is the fact that it creates inequity based on employment and financial status. It allows those with money, or with good jobs that provide private health insurance, to have access to both the public services and the private practices. Meanwhile, those with less income, or jobs that do not provide insurance benefits, can only access the public service. This inequity is well understood to be a significant determinant of health and illness in a society that discriminates against the poor. That is why the Canadian health care system, if the integrity of its principles was being fully protected, is a more socially just and more effective model than a two-tiered system.

It is important that we begin to look at this discrepancy and make all such health services (e.g., counselling and psychotherapy) equitably accessible to all members of the public. This may involve a variety of approaches, such as sweeping all private practitioners into the public system, or allowing private practitioners to bill the public health system for services provided to clients without money or insurance. It is hard to claim that we have a client-centered system when the overall structure itself (two-tiered) actively discriminates against some of our clients (the public) based on money.

Actions for system managers and leaders:

Begin discussions with government about ways of eliminating the discriminatory impact of having this two-tiered system, to help ensure equal access to mental health care for all citizens.

Actions for clients, supporters, and advocates:

Advocate with government to find ways to address this inequity.

CHAPTER 4

KEEPING HEALTHY PEOPLE HEALTHY

It is commonly argued that a key reason for long wait times for mental health and addiction programs is that they are under-resourced. They don't have enough staff or money. Well, it isn't that simple and the statement isn't necessarily valid in all cases. If your house is too small for the amount of stuff you have, you can either get a bigger house (more resource/capacity), or you can reduce the amount of stuff you have, or reduce the amount of new stuff you bring into the house.

When looking at any situation in which capacity is not adequate to meet demand, both sides of the equation need to be considered. Under-resourced, under-funded, and other such common terms are not absolute. They are *relative* terms. In other words, they don't mean anything unless we are comparing things to one another. There is no absolute right amount of services. It is all about comparison between how much service we need to meet the demand and how much service we have to offer. To simply say we need more is only reflecting one side of the issue. Of course, the point here is that our system typically has not made a focused effort to reduce the demand on services. Imagine for a minute that fewer people needed help. We would therefore not need as much money or staffing, or at least we would not be saying we need more.

The issue of being under-funded or under-resourced can be addressed either by (1) providing more services, or (2) creating less need for the services. Typically, the entire focus of our system has been on the first alternative. Because the system is designed within this psychiatric, pathology-oriented paradigm, the second alternative has rarely, if ever, even been considered by those leading the mental health system. The traditional model is designed to provide treatment of illness, so this other preventative, demand-reduction work has just not been acknowledged or understood.

While this may appear to be criticism of the leadership of mental health and addictions, the oversight/limitation is not actually their fault. The training of those who have been running most of these programs is almost entirely clinical. Their background is in the assessment and treatment of illness. Their education, training, and experience have not provided them with the knowledge or skills in evidence-based demand-reduction work. It has not taught them about prevention and health promotion. It is exactly the same as noting that someone trained in health promotion and prevention is not trained to think clinically. A health promoter has a specialty skill set that a clinician does not, and vice-versa. Neither is better nor worse, or more or less important. We each simply come from the limited frame of reference that our education and experience give us, and those limitations often determine what our focus and abilities will or will not be.

There are a couple main ways to approach this goal of reducing demand on the system within a client-centered framework. One is for us to get better at keeping healthy people healthy, so they don't require any clinical type of service. This would involve using methods that are non-clinical, evidence-based, and suited to the needs of that healthy population (client-centered). The second is to be more effective at providing early intervention supports to reduce the number of people requiring the more-intensive and more-expensive therapeutic and medical services. These would be non-therapeutic, but supportive, and would help healthy people who are experiencing risk factors or early symptoms. These also would be designed specifically to meet the unique preventative needs of that population (client-centered).

Going back to our former discussion, the more we do at the early end of the continuum, or on the lower levels of the tiered model, the more we will be able to maintain or increase capacity to meet demand at the intensive, upper levels. In other words, if we are better at meeting the needs of *all* clients across the continuum, not just those with identifiable symptoms of disorders, we can improve our capacity and meet the demand better by having fewer people who end up needing mental illness care.

Health Promotion and Healthy Public Policy

Many of the things that cause us to be healthy or ill are related to the social, economic, and physical environments we live in. They are often referred to as the determinants of health. Many of those determinants not only have an impact on our physical health, but also influence people's mental health and substance use. For example, we are well beyond wondering if anxiety or depression can be caused and/or exacerbated by not having sufficient income to support the essential things in life. We know it can. We are well beyond wondering if financial status and psychological well-being are affected by a person's level of literacy and education. We know they are. It is no longer a question whether unhealthy processed food (more affordable than healthy food) contributes to the incidence of chronic disease, which in turn is strongly related to the experience of depression. We know this. These are but a few examples of the connections between these broad population variables and the experience of mental illness and addiction problems. This means that we can reduce the incidence or severity of mental illness and addictions by addressing some of those population-level factors. We can reduce the demand on the services that we say are overburdened and underfunded.

Even if we get down to what appear to be individual-level determinants of health, often referred to as personal health practices, the *solutions* are not necessarily at the individual level. Take alcohol and tobacco-use as examples. We have known for a very long time that rates of smoking were significantly influenced by the behaviours of 'Big Tobacco' (Big Tobacco refers to the handful of large tobacco companies that control the industry globally). The tobacco industry became a master at the art of influencing entire populations to take up smoking. It became a master at targeting children and adolescents, while keeping it hard for anyone to notice it or prove it. For decades, without us knowing that was happening, we continued to believe that simply educating our young people about the risks and harms of smoking would keep them away from cigarettes. That individual focus, and reliance on education, is now known to be ineffective. As a result, many years of educating left us consistently losing the battle, and our children, to tobacco.

The tide began to turn on Big Tobacco when a public policy approach was taken, and regulation of the industry itself became the focus. These measures included eliminating advertising, continually increasing price, preventing people from being exposed to smoke unwillingly, making tobacco products less available, and enforcing age limits for purchasing. This approach sparked new trends in the *next* generation who would otherwise have been influenced by the industry, the same as their parents and grandparents before them. This type of population-focused health promotion, using public policy, is almost always about normalizing or de-normalizing a behaviour in the next and future generations. As a result of this approach, Nova Scotia alone has more than 100,000 fewer smokers than it did 15 years ago. Given that we only have about 1,000,000 people, that is a significant reduction on demand for addiction treatment and for hospital care for cancer, heart disease, and respiratory illness.

We are now seeing the same tactics in the alcohol industry that were used by tobacco. 'Big Alcohol' is using these methods to promote increased drinking, and to normalize it among children and adolescents. This is evident in the kinds of advertisements we see. Look at who is depicted in them, what the themes are, or when they are placed on television. If you drink a certain brand of alcohol, you will suddenly have many beautiful women wanting you sexually. If you drink a certain kind of beer, you will have a cabin by a lake, a bunch of half-naked friends dancing around a fire, a nice car in the driveway, and no worries in the world.

These ads are clearly targeting naive and vulnerable adolescents in our society, not adults. Children and adolescents are being exposed to great amounts of advertising influence that we know causes them to drink earlier and more. As with tobacco, we know that educating our kids to make individual choices not to drink, or to drink less, is not the answer.

79

It is ineffective. Education does not prevent substance use/abuse. It is important for our young people to learn about harmful substances, but it does not change behaviour. It is necessary but not sufficient. Regulation of the industry through public policy is the answer, as it was with tobacco.

The international evidence is clear (Babor, Caetano, Casswell, Edwards, & Geisbrecht, 2010). We need to stop our children from being exposed to alcohol advertising. We need to use price as a way of reducing the per capita level of consumption of alcohol. We need to restrict the type of advertising used (e.g., using hyper-sexualization or the expected attainment of a desirable lifestyle to promote drinking). Finally, we need to make alcohol products less available. This is not a recommendation for prohibition, but for recognizing that this substance causes or contributes to breast cancer (and at least four other types), heart disease, injuries, sexual assaults, and domestic violence. We should not be pretending alcohol is an ordinary commodity, allowing the industry's profit motive to harm our children and send them looking for treatment in our programs. An evidence-based approach to reducing the demand on our mental health and addiction programs would be to take these regulatory actions. A client-centered approach would also be to use our legislative powers to keep our children (the client) healthy, rather than knowingly allow them to be harmed by the industry and then provide them with treatment services for their cancer, heart disease, or addiction.

As we enter legalization of cannabis in Canada, we need to learn from our historical failures and more recent successes with tobacco, and from our abysmal failure at protecting our children from the alcohol industry. We need to apply the same lessons because all three of these industries will always have a singular profit motive. They will also have a primary target of children and adolescents because they are the main (if not only) source of new, lifetime customers. We need to legalize it, but specifically for the purpose of public health. That means we completely ignore the industry, do not consult with it in the creation of regulations, and thereby do not support the industry in its profit goals. Our job as a society, and the primary purpose for legalization, is to protect the public health and in particular our youth. The evidence from our experience and research with tobacco and alcohol is clear. We know it requires that there be no advertising of any kind because its only purpose is increasing sales. Why would we allow the promotion of increased use of a substance that is far from harmless? We know it requires that there be no sales anywhere except in a government-owned monopoly distribution system, and a strictly-enforced age limit (later than adolescence) to purchase. The list goes on. A good review of this topic was published by the Center for Addiction and Mental Health (Jean-François Crépault; Centre for Addiction and Mental Health, 2014), and another by the Canadian Centre on Substance Abuse (Canadian Centre on Substance Abuse, 2015)

If we learn from tobacco, and adopt the kind of tight restrictions for cannabis that have effectively reduced smoking, we will be preventing addiction, schizophrenia, and other illnesses in the next generation. If we adopt our completely-inept approach to alcohol, we will create more of these illnesses than ever imagined, and it is our children and grandchildren who will suffer. If we think we can legalize cannabis, use loose regulation of the industry, allow easy and open production, access, and advertising, and then educate our way into healthy children with bright futures, we are mistaken. Education simply and unequivocally does not work to prevent substance use. It is necessary but not sufficient. It affects knowledge but not behaviour. We are decades past knowing that fact. Failing to learn from the past leaves us repeating the same mistakes.

Let's look at these issues of regulation of tobacco, alcohol, and cannabis in the context of the client-centered theme of this book. Our public is the client of our health system. Our public is the client of our mental health and addiction programs. These drug industries (tobacco, alcohol, or cannabis) are not the client. Yet, for decades, elected officials have avoided regulating them according to what the evidence says is best for the well-being of the public. We have an industry-centered approach to public policy in this regard. By virtue of allowing alcohol companies to advertise insidiously to children, we are determining the interest of the industry to be a higher priority than the health of the children (our client). If we allow the cannabis industry to influence the way we regulate its own activities, rather than unequivocally implementing a regulatory framework solely designed to protect our children and public, we will be taking an industry-centered approach. We will not be taking a client-centered approach because the industry is not our client and therefore its interests cannot be considered above the health of the public.

Now back to the determinants of health. Even the determinant of health that refers most directly to individual behavior (personal health practices) relies on healthy public policy to influence it in a positive way. While educating people doesn't work, regulation of industries that produce harmful products does work. If we want to reduce the demand on mental health and addiction services, we need to engage directly in creating public policy that is client-centered, not industry-centered.

When we talk about the health of a population, and the work of government and its public organizations to ensure the well-being of that population, we must step out of our individual focus. We must recognize that, in this case, the population is the client and improving and maintaining the mental health of that population is the job. It is not about individuals. It is about changing the environment in which an entire population lives in order to promote and protect its overall health status. The client might be a community that is experiencing increased drinking rates because of a new alcohol retail store being opened. As community members start to become concerned, watching their family members, neighbors, and young people experience more alcohol-related problems, that community as a whole really can be seen as the client. It needs service. But, the service needed to meet the needs of that particular client is public policy, through reducing the unnecessarily high level of availability of alcohol, and closing that local store. Keep alcohol reasonably accessible but a little less convenient to get.

Some people have looked at this health promotion work at the far left of the continuum as being just fluff. They falsely believe it is merely an education task, and certainly not something that is worth our time or money because it does not produce outcomes. People have difficulty thinking beyond the individual level, and even more difficulty accepting the fact that behaviour-change in populations rarely, if ever, is influenced by information/education alone.

It's not that hard to understand if we think about our own lives. Let's take a food example, and look at it through two questions: Do you think most people in Canada know that foods high in sodium, sugar, and fat cause illness and disease? Of course they do. When I ask my university classes if they know this, they all raise their hands – 100%. Now, among all those people who know this information, do many of them still eat those foods? Of course they do. When I ask my university students if they eat such foods, about 75% raise their hands, right after acknowledging that they are aware of the facts.

There are many aspects of health promotion that can be addressed through public policy, and that can help maintain well-being in our population in the areas of mental health and addictions. These include the substance use examples already described. They include occupational health and safety legislation that guarantees people the right to have a workplace free of verbally and emotionally abusive behaviour. They include legislation and regulations that protect people's human rights and prevent discrimination or oppression. There are many. Some are simple and obvious, and others are complex and multi-systemic.

Let's look at a current example in which different components of public policy jointly have direct effects on mental health and demand on the mental health system. In recent years, there have been very-high-profile sexual assault cases in Canada. Not surprisingly, in many such cases we have seen victims not being believed, either at the investigative level, or in court. In one such case in Nova Scotia, a young woman, Rehtaeh Parsons, tragically ended her own life as a result of the sequence of events following her assault. The result of such a case is an insidious message to victims, that coming forward and reporting sexual assault is futile and will only harm oneself. What we have is a public institution, the criminal justice system, operating on policies and procedures that may be inadvertently causing more trauma to women. It is causing those who are sexually assaulted (which we know to be most often but certainly not exclusively women) to stay quiet and suffer in silence. It is causing people who are victimized to experience deeper levels of depression, anxiety, and post-traumatic stress disorder than might otherwise exist.

The prevention of these psychological illnesses in that population can be addressed through changes in public policy. Fewer sexual assault survivors will need intensive therapy if they are heard, supported, taken seriously, and not re-victimized through victim-blaming. But, to achieve this, we need changes in the criminal justice system (public policy) so people feel safe coming forward. In other words, we need a client-centered approach that designs criminal justice policy around the needs of that unique population of sexual assault survivors. This is yet another example of how improving the socio-political environment in which we live, through public policy, can reduce demand on the mental health and addiction system.

The bottom line is that if we want to reduce the demand on our services, we need to apply science. We must advocate for evidence-based public policy that puts the well-being of our public first. We need to address regulation of industries that produce addictive and harmful substances, and we must do so with health as the priority over industry or even government revenue. We need to correct social injustices that cause harm to vulnerable people. We need, as part of our mandate in the public mental health and addiction system, the job of openly advocating for such changes because it is our job to prevent mental illness and addictions. This would be an evidence-based method of doing so. We need our governments to give us this mandate to serve as expert advisors on healthy public policy, not just on the usual and limited clinical service delivery issues.

This is one important way to address the demand side of the capacity/ demand equation in our struggling system. This is one important way to provide client-centered service to all the healthy people whom we are supposed to keep healthy.

Actions for system managers and leaders:

Learn about healthy public policy and its preventative effects on our future potential clients, and incorporate this knowledge into your daily work and your advocacy opportunities as they arise.

Actions for clients, supporters, and advocates:

1. Advocate assertively for strict regulation of the alcohol industry, based on evidence referenced here, for the sake of protecting your children and grandchildren.

2. Advocate assertively for strict regulation of the cannabis industry, based on evidence referenced here, for the sake of protecting your children and grandchildren.

3. Advocate for a population-focused effort to address the key determinants of health, as discussed.

Health Promotion and Prevention in Schools

For years, our attempts to do prevention work in schools has been based on completely ineffective methods, as discussed elsewhere in this book. We have spent our time and money trying to use fear/scare tactics to explain to students all the bad things that can happen if they use drugs, for instance. We have tried providing information and rational arguments about why children shouldn't bully or hurt one another, or shouldn't try smoking. In the vast majority of health behaviours, these two approaches do not work.

More recently, we have learned that there is preventative impact in social and emotional learning during childhood. Many programs have been developed and a couple examples of such programs which have demonstrated effectiveness are Promoting Alternative Thinking Strategies – "PATHS" (SEAK, 2013), and The Good Behaviour Game – "PAX" (Embry, 2016). These programs have demonstrated remarkable preventative impacts on substance use, mental illness, and socially aggressive behaviour, while improving empathy and even enhancing academic performance. It is important to note that these are not just in-class curricular programs, but rather involve all school staff, and ideally parents, in a culture shift and an adoption of a new approach to how language is used with the children to support the learning.

Our only problem is that the uptake and implementation of these programs is slow or non-existent across our school systems. This is such an odd situation. Here we are with an evidence-based way to reduce the number of young people who end up experiencing mental illness or addiction problems, and many of our mental health programs have not recognized this as their role. They have not engaged with the school systems and co-sponsored and co-funded the adoption of such programs. Again this reflects the limited perspective of a system built on a medical, pathology-oriented model. If we took an approach that served *all* of our clients (the public), we would be implementing such evidence-based prevention methods across our school systems. That would keep healthy people healthy, reduce demand on the mental health and addiction system, and make us question our constant call for needing more money and resources.

Actions for system managers and leaders:

Contact your local education system and begin a partnership to achieve complete implementation of a proven social and emotional learning program, such as PATHS or the PAX Good Behaviour Game, to protect our children from preventable problems, and to reduce demand on our treatment services.

Actions for clients, supporters, and advocates:

Contact your local school system, and also your local mental health and addiction systems, either at the community level or at the government level, and advocate for the adoption of one of these programs across the whole education system in your area. This will help keep your children and your grandchildren healthy with less chance of their needing help from a mental health and addiction treatment program.

CHAPTER 5

EARLY INTERVENTION TO PREVENT ILLNESS

The previous chapter lays out approaches to keeping healthy people from ever needing any direct care from a mental health and addiction program. It was about creating a healthy population. That is one way to reduce demand on our mental illness-care programs. The second way to address the demand component of this apparent misfit between our resources and the pressures placed upon them is early intervention to prevent small problems from becoming big problems. While the previous chapter was about keeping healthy people healthy, here we are talking about keeping early or minor symptoms or challenges from becoming illness.

As noted earlier, the mental health system has generally not been inclusive of this type of early-intervention support work. This is likely the result of a few key variables.

First, as previously noted, the leadership in mental health and addiction programs has been comprised almost exclusively of clinicians who move up through the program into management. They have spent their careers seeing things from a clinical perspective, so their predisposition is to focus on and maintain psychotherapeutic work as the exclusive mandate of the program. This is an understandable manifestation of the type of education and career experience that has formed their knowledge base and their perspective. It is how they have been trained to see this field.

Secondly, it is possible that the lack of attention to early intervention for mild-to-moderate concerns has been the result of attempts to manage capacity. For example, if you have 100 people looking for service, and you believe you can only serve 10, then moving the cut-off line by redefining inclusion criteria can help you achieve the inclusion of only the 10. In other words, focus your efforts on the most serious, and anyone not meeting that definition is excluded. Your program is therefore not failing to meet the demand. Instead, it is simply defining what it does and does not treat. Phrases like "We can't be all things to all people." are often used to help justify or rationalize such inclusion/ exclusion criteria. That's great rationalization, but system leaders who take this approach are assuming they have the right to exclude entire segments of the taxpaying public (the client) – which, in a public service, they do not.

In addition, there is some of what I call *professional elitism* involved in the system's avoidance of early intervention work. Professional elitism is used here to describe a sense that some types of professions, training, positons, etc., are better, smarter, or more important than others in the system. If we consider the nature of the need at that early intervention and support level, we would recognize that it is typically below the expertise and skill level of highly-trained clinicians. If we want to utilize resources properly, by matching scope of practice to scope of need, some of this early intervention work would require paraprofessionals who have been trained in basic counselling skills. It would be an inappropriate use of public money and staff to have this work done by psychiatrists, clinical psychologists, etc., because it is not a medical or psychotherapeutic need or task. It is preventative, supportive, early intervention counselling. If we recognize that a client-centered system must serve those clients who are in need of such early supportive services, and not simply exclude them, then we must consider the best kind of skills and staffing for this role. There is a big gap in the system that can best be filled by paraprofessional trained counsellors (i.e., people trained in counselling not therapy, and who are not registered as clinical psychologists, social workers, psychiatrists, registered counselling therapists, etc.).

Unfortunately, many of the clinicians who have found themselves in leadership roles struggle with this concept and are averse to the idea because of a variety of arguments that don't really stand up under scrutiny. They will say we should only hire people who are accountable to a regulatory body that registers or licenses a type of profession. That way, if the employee does something wrong, she can be held accountable. However, as an employee, she can still be held accountable by her employer without the need for any such external licensing body. Some of the leaders will say that people who are not trained and regulated as professionals pose risks related to ethical conduct. Many of us who have worked in this field, however, have seen more than our share of unethical behaviour from licensed professionals as well. It is a staff-management issue that applies to all employees. Our failure to manage inappropriate conduct in professional and paraprofessional employees is a completely separate problem. A staff person being registered or licenced in no way prevents unethical conduct. That is about the person, not the professional designation.

If we are building a truly client-centered service, then we make decisions that match resources to the needs of the client, regardless of our own professional biases and preferences, and regardless of our aversion to holding staff accountable. Providing paraprofessional counsellors for early intervention, supportive counselling would be a client-centered service because it is designed to match the type of service to the needs of the person being served. Unfortunately, the resistance to such hiring, due to professional elitism, may be a barrier to doing appropriate early intervention work.

Substance use and many areas of mental illness are progressive, which in this case is a bad thing. It means they keep getting worse if unaddressed. Given that this is the way many physical illnesses work, this should not be a surprise. If support and intervention are not available early for hypertension, type 2 diabetes, depression, or frequent drinking, the people experiencing those symptoms will undoubtedly find themselves requiring hospitalization and treatment for stroke, ketoacedosis, suicide watch, or alcohol overdose or dependence. If the only service we provide is acute care, which has traditionally been the case for all of our health care system (including mental health), then there is no opportunity to change the vector that people are on. There is no point at which the person's course of *potential* illness is interrupted with anything resembling either primary or secondary prevention. Problems develop and progress until they are severe enough to justify engaging with the acute care system or, in this case, the mental illness treatment system. In other words, we let them get worse until they meet the inclusion criteria – being ill.

For mental health and addictions, we need to build in mechanisms to facilitate people engaging in early support in order to prevent that progression to illness. Creating those mechanisms is both the opportunity and the challenge. The one area where there has perhaps been the greatest momentum across Nova Scotia and elsewhere in Canada in recent years is the insertion of mental health and addiction clinical staff into collaborative practice in primary health care clinics. In other words, there has been a move to put clinicians into the family doctors' offices.

This accomplishes a couple key things. It facilitates conversations with clients about their substance use and/or mental health issues when they perhaps had not been giving attention to those issues before, or would not have seen them as requiring attention. It also helps build greater capacity by enhancing comfort level among doctors and nurse practitioners in dealing with these types of issues. All of that contributes to earlier intervention, and less stigma. Perhaps most important of all is the fact that this approach is client-centered. This is about bringing services to where the clients are anyway, without requiring them to self-identify and take the leap to contact a mental health and addiction program. People are comfortable going to their doctor or nurse practitioner. If these other health issues can also be addressed in the same context, then we are essentially making the system fit the client. We are reducing the aversion that comes with stigma, and thereby making it easier for clients to get help earlier, before they are ill. This is client-centered service. This same client-centered approach needs to be replicated in other settings and other kinds of situations.

Let's take another look at the earlier-mentioned issue of sexual assault. We previously considered how public policy change in the criminal justice system could reduce demand for mental health and addiction services. Now, consider what a client-centered approach to early intervention would look like in terms of the public mental health and addiction system.

There is no question that sexual assault is among the most traumatic events a person can experience. As a result, survivors of an assault invariably experience psychological distress. This would most commonly take the form of depression, anxiety, and post-traumatic stress disorder, and often substance abuse and addiction as a method of self-medicating those feelings. The nature of these kinds of symptoms, behaviours, and illnesses is that they are all progressive. Again, that means if they are untreated, they will most often get worse over time.

In a traditional psychiatric paradigm, these early experiences of sadness, stress, fear, paranoia, guilt, shame, self-isolation, etc., would be considered non-pathological and would not commonly be treated. At such an early stage, they don't usually represent a diagnosable disorder. Therefore, people experiencing such problems may remain excluded from the service, or be made to wait based on the way in which cases are prioritized. This approach, as previously discussed, may not be surprising in the context of the pathology-oriented way the culture of programs has evolved.

Any conditions or sets of symptoms that are progressive are naturally occurring opportunities for prevention of more serious illness. Simply put, the earlier the progression of such symptoms is interrupted, the less likely they will become severe and chronic later on. We have come to accept this idea in the case of physical illness. We all know that early detection of cancer increases our ability to stop its progression. We know that early identification of rising blood pressure or rising blood-glucose levels can allow for either medical or lifestyle interventions that often reverse, or at least stop, the progression of these symptoms into hypertension or diabetes.

In these cases, our primary care and acute care systems take such early detection and prevention quite seriously. People are encouraged to seek early assessment or help for such concerns, and the appropriate prevention and early intervention services are made available when such cases arise. It is seen as a priority in many cases (e.g., cancer) because of the benefit it can have for both the patient and the health care system. Mental health and addiction issues should be no different. Prevention and early intervention are essential to the well-being of our top priority, the client, and essential to the transformation and sustainability of the mental health and addiction system.

Now, let's get back to the sexual assault example. In a common sexual assault scenario, a person who has been assaulted shows up at the emergency department of a local hospital. The survivor's medical needs are attended to as the first course of action.

In many areas, working from a traditional model, while the medical and forensic part of the process is carried out at the hospital, the mental health part is a secondary step. The survivor is either provided with a telephone number to call, in order to speak with a therapist about the trauma, or a referral form is completed by the nurse and sent to the mental health and addiction program. From the perspective of a client-centered, preventative early-intervention approach, there are several problems with this.

First, simply giving the client a phone number and leaving this traumatized person to have to make a call to strangers and give the reason for the call is a perfect recipe for a person not ever reaching out for help. Between the anxiety and the self/societally-inflicted sense of shame, this is an inappropriate expectation to place on this person. Second, in either approach, the survivor ends up having to go meet with a complete stranger and re-tell some of the story. Finally, if this happens in an area that has long wait times, we miss an opportunity to intervene early enough to prevent further harm and chronic illness. We are left with a typical case of someone going from needing moderate support, counselling, and skill building, to someone needing intensive and longer-term psychotherapeutic or medical intervention. We would have allowed the person to progress to the point of meeting our inclusion criteria.

What would a client-centered mental health response to sexual assault look like? Let's start at the emergency department again. If we had a case of an attempted suicide, the medical team and the mental health team would both be involved early. If a case of heart failure showed up, a cardiologist might be called to be part of the care from the beginning.

With sexual assault, we already know ahead of time the major factors that are important for the health system to address, including medical care, forensic evidence collection, and psychological care. There is no reason all those resources can't be mobilized concurrently from the beginning, as we do with other situations. In such a system, when the survivor shows up identifying an assault, the appropriate members of the health care team would all be called in at once. These would include the nurse or physician who will be doing the medical and forensic components, and a mental health counsellor/clinician who will be starting to provide the support needed. In an unobtrusive way, this clinician can begin to build trust and rapport just by being there, listening, comforting, reassuring, helping fend off harmful self-blaming attributions, etc.

The benefits of this approach are many. The medical professional can focus on the medical issues and evidence-collection processes, and know that the patient's emotional needs are being supported. The survivor would have someone there who has no purpose except to be supportive. The survivor ends up with someone in the mental health program who already knows the basic story and, therefore, does not need any of it repeated if there is a later counselling or therapy session. The survivor has someone able to directly coordinate and arrange easy access to whatever kinds of mental health supports or services are needed or wanted, and ensure good linkage with any and all available community support resources. If the survivor has family or friends present, they also end up with a mental health contact person, with whom they have built at least some initial rapport and trust, and who can help serve as a navigator for them in a complex system. Simply put, this is a client-centered approach that is primarily focused on preventing the development or progression of trauma-related mental illness or substance use. This is preventative early intervention at its best.

This is taking the services to meet and support the client where s/he is, rather than sitting and waiting in case the client reaches out later. This requires having no exclusion criteria that would get in the way of such an immediate early-intervention service.

If the sexual assault survivor was your sister or son, how would you want the system to work? Would you want the physical issues addressed and then have your loved one wait for a phone call for a mental health appointment? Would you want your loved one to have to take a phone number and make a call to a stranger and start all over again? Would you want your family member to experience worsening symptoms and end up with significant depression or post-traumatic stress disorder because of no early support available? Of course not. You would want your loved one treated as a whole person, with the system providing all that is needed to keep that person whole and healthy from the beginning.

In sexual assault services, the survivor is offered the opportunity to have the forensic evidence collected (i.e., rape kit) for potential criminal proceedings. In areas still using an older model, police would be called in if the survivor said yes to having the kit completed, and they would begin gathering information to proceed with investigation and/or charges. In a client-centered approach, however, the survivor would be clearly told there is no statute of limitations on sexual assault, so there is no rush to decide about pressing charges. S/he would be told that the kit could be done at that time without needing to have any interaction with police and without having to press charges. Then months or years later, if s/he decided to proceed with charges, s/he could. This way, the client is the one in charge of every step that is or is not taken.

This complete freedom to decide to collect the evidence, with absolutely no obligation to interact with police or commit to charges, is crucial. From a mental health perspective, one thing a survivor needs to be given, above all else, is control. This is not just an issue of evidence and the criminal justice system. It is both symbolically and tangibly a process of trying to help the survivor regain some of the control s/he had lost as a result of the sexual assault. This client-centered approach can contribute to our prevention and early intervention goals, therefore, by starting to re-empower the survivor and interrupt the progression of any perceived helplessness that may have started developing. In other words, the way we design our processes for the emergency department and the police can also help prevent a sexual assault survivor from developing more-chronic problems later that require intensive and longer-term therapy. Achieving this requires good interagency partnerships, which are discussed in a later chapter.

There are many such situations in which we have the ability to provide early intervention and support to prevent illness, or at least prevent progression from mild/moderate challenges to more severe and persistent disorders. A few program examples of client-centered early intervention are described in detail in a later chapter. The suggested paradigm shift from the psychiatric, pathology-oriented model to a client-centered system, allows for and in fact requires that such early-intervention work be incorporated and emphasized as a *dominant* component of the system. Clients at all levels of struggle, symptomatology, and illness deserve to receive service that matches their level of need. It is easily argued that those with the least-severe problems (candidates for early intervention supports) are the most important segment of our client population if we are concerned about sustainability of the public system. Such clients require less-intensive services, for a shorter duration, and have the greatest potential to maintain or regain a high level of health/functionality and not require service in future. Demand on the system is thereby reduced, and we are able to manage within existing resources.

Actions for system managers and leaders:

1. Begin to shift resources toward preventative early intervention, as opportunities arise. When a clinical position becomes vacant, hire someone trained to do early intervention supportive counselling and skill-building, rather than a therapist, and start seeing people who are not yet ill. This will begin to gradually reduce the demand for therapy.

2. At the same time, start identifying those clients who would usually have been scheduled to see a therapist, but who really need less-intensive support, and schedule them with counsellors. They are better suited to the client's need for lower-intensity, early-intervention counselling and support, and because they cost less, this approach also happens to use public dollars more efficiently (thereby freeing up money for increasing capacity).

Actions for clients, supporters, and advocates:

1. Seek help early, and don't wait until you have a serious illness, whether the system seems to be ready for that or not. This is one way to help system leaders start to see the need for early intervention counselling.

2. Do not get caught up in the myth that you need to see a psychiatrist, as many people believe, or even a clinical psychologist, clinical social worker, or therapist. Just ask for someone to talk with, get in earlier as a result (especially if the program in your area is progressive and has easily-accessible counselling), and then together you can figure out if you need more of a specialty service.

Demand Reduction Summary

In these last two chapters, we have discussed in depth the idea and methods of reducing the demand on our treatment services. This is a major shift. We simply cannot expect to improve access and quality of care in our mental health and addiction system unless we shake off the ways of the past and start focusing on reducing the demand for these mental-illness-care services. This is not a new idea. Health promotion specialists have known it for decades. It is, however, an idea that has never been embraced by the mental health system leadership.

This lack of movement from concept to practice is directly the result of the system operating within a medicalized model. This psychiatric paradigm is not designed to incorporate health promotion or early intervention. The people trained to be experts in the assessment, diagnosis, and treatment of psychological and psychiatric disorders are just that – they are experts in one component of the work. They are experts in one end of the continuum. They are experts in the upper levels of the tiered model. We need them to be exactly what they are, and do exactly what they do. But, it is insufficient for our public system to *only* do that part of the work, *only* use professionals with that specific but limited training and education, and *only* serve that small segment of our client population (the public).

I recall sitting in a meeting of senior leaders in the mental health and addiction system, and talking about what will be the priorities of that leadership group for the upcoming couple years. As the term prevention was bantered around by all, I continued only to hear examples and language that meant clinical intervention. It struck me as an odd, shared misuse and misunderstanding of the term among so many intelligent people. I recall weighing in on the issues by suggesting that evidence-based health promotion was part of our necessary mandate. I gave examples of how we should be advising and advocating with government about specific public policy issues, such as regulating and reducing the alcohol industry's level of advertising to children and adolescents. I was shocked to hear, from a senior and prominent psychiatrist, a combination of confusion in understanding the concept and resistance to our being involved in such work. His response was along the lines of "Why would we do that? That is not our job. Our job is providing treatment services." This is a prime example of how our system has been led by, and framed within, a paradigm limited by pathology-oriented thinking. Such expertise and thinking is clearly necessary, but needs to be moved from being the overall model that governs the *whole* system, to being a specialized component of service within a *broader* client-centered model.

This concept of starting to focus on demand reduction is not exclusive to mental health and addictions. We know that our public health care resources in Canada have struggled to keep up with demand. Costs have continued to grow. All the while, we sit back and keep waiting for people to get sick and come to our doctors and nurses to be fixed. All the while, we continue to embrace the medical-model approach that is based on the limited viewpoint of those who are only trained to treat illness. We still put very little effort into evidence-based health promotion that can reduce the demand on the system. The medical paradigm doesn't allow for it. For example, we avoid using Federal regulation to reduce sodium in processed foods, and instead we wait and treat high blood pressure and strokes caused by that sodium, and put stents in people's arteries.

We know, however, that if we use health-oriented public policy supported by social marketing, we can reduce the number of people developing heart disease, cancer, respiratory illness, and type 2 diabetes. We also know that such health promotion and early intervention can reduce demand on our mental health and addiction system. We just need to stop thinking through a medicalized paradigm, and stop thinking our job is to serve only *some* of our clients (those with established illness). We must start recognizing that the healthy members of our taxpaying public are also our clients, and those experiencing challenges or early symptoms of what might be illness someday are also our clients. We need to adopt a client-centered approach that ensures the overall system is guided by people with expertise in everything from health promotion to early intervention, to psychotherapy, to psychiatry, not merely by those who have an important, but limited specialty at one end of the continuum.

We would never entertain the idea that the leadership of mental health and addiction programs be exclusively controlled by health promoters. It would make no sense because the specialty treatment services wouldn't be well enough understood, and would potentially be neglected or undervalued. The opposite is what we have now. We have a system exclusively controlled by people trained at one end of the continuum.

A client-centered paradigm allows for all such specialties, allows for all of our public (the clients) to be served appropriately, and allows us to reduce demand on the strained mental health and addiction system. Back to my earlier analogy, if our house is too small for the amount of stuff we have, we can either keep trying to build a bigger house, or we can reduce how much stuff we bring in. If we serve our whole public properly, we reduce how much stuff we bring into our house, allowing more room for the stuff that really needs to be there.

CHAPTER 6

Helping Clients Contact the System Easily

The next few chapters introduce some of the practical ways to apply the client-centered paradigm to particular components of a public mental health and addiction system. They describe approaches that can help make the system less like a castle, with a moat around it, that people can't access. Specifically, the present chapter considers a client's navigation to the first encounter he has with the program. How does he find the program and contact it? How do we help that contact take place, and what kind of experience will it be for the client? What should the processes look like at that first point of contact in a client-centered paradigm?

Single-Door Entry Point

What does a client want and need? Simplicity, I would suggest. If the client were your sister, what kind of access system would you want her to have?

Most people are very clear when answering such a question. They do not want to search through multiple phone numbers to figure out which one they need to call. They do not want to call one number, only to be told they need to call a different one. They do not want to have one way to access mental health and another for addictions. If they are dealing with *both* mental health *and* addiction problems, they don't consider themselves as divided into these separate parts. We must make sure there is a single phone number for people to use to make contact, and that the number is listed everywhere possible (e.g., organization website, phone directories, websites of partner organizations, patient-orientation packages, posters or handouts in hospitals, schools, posts on social media).

Over the decades, one of the barriers to this single access point has been the technical limitations on having one telephone number for a geographically-large, multi-site program, as is the case in both rural and urban areas. However, we are fortunate that this is no longer a reason to have multiple contact numbers. Sometimes the phone system itself will cost more money to set up, but this is an important part of the client-access experience. Its level of importance further increases if we consider the vulnerable state some clients are in when seeking help. In this state, many people's thoughts, feelings, anxiety are such that they diminish patience, tolerance for complicated, multi-step processes, and determination and perseverance to continue trying to gain access. Consequently, if our system doesn't make the initial contact smooth and simple, many clients will not access service because it feels, or truly is, too difficult.

Actions for system managers and leaders:

1. Create a simple and singular method of clients finding how to make contact, such as a single phone number.

2. Advertise it everywhere, and make sure especially that all other health care providers (e.g., primary care doctors, nurses on the medical units) are aware of that single entry point.

Actions for clients, supporters, and advocates:

If in your area, it is not clear where to go, or there are too many options and no information about which one is for which purpose, advocate for that to be changed. Let your health system leaders, and government officials, know that there needs to be a simple, single phone number, so the client does not need to figure out the structure of the whole system in order to make contact.

Any Door is the Right Door

Initially, this may seem to conflict with the previous argument that we need a single entry point. It doesn't. It is an add-on. From a client perspective, it is still very important to have one central method of accessing services, without the confusion of multiple numbers, locations, or program streams to figure out. However, what about a person who ends up making contact in a different way? Let's explore how that should be handled.

A client shows up at a mental health and addiction satellite office that is not the program's primary, single-entry point. What should happen? Start with the key question again. If the client were your spouse, how would you want that process to be handled? In a rigid, single-entry-point system, what might happen is that the client would be given the main phone number and directed to go home and call that number to begin the process of accessing service. Is that what you would want for your wife if she made a trip to the clinic in person looking for access? Probably not. If there is a staff person at the community office who is capable of doing *the intake* (the same thing that would be done if a person phoned in), you would probably prefer to have it done right there and then, in person. It would show respect for the fact that your wife drove in. More importantly, it would avoid giving this client another step to take, or another hoop to jump through, just to meet the system's sometimes-dogmatic need for administrative standardization. Even if the only staff person in the office is a clinician, who has a client to see, he could possibly even make the call to the intake staff, and allow the client to complete the intake over the phone right there at the satellite office. At least the client then gets what she came for.

In a truly client-centered approach, any door is the right door. We may create and promote a single-access point, but we must remain prepared to be flexible in responding to clients. If one makes an attempt to access help, but doesn't do it in quite the way we want her to, she should not be punished for that. It is the responsibility of the program and its staff to accept inconvenience to avoid the client experiencing it. That responsibility involves making the process easy for the client. It means being responsive and not expecting everything to fit neatly into a specific administrative box. It means welcoming that client wherever and whenever she makes contact, and doing the work to get her into the services she needs. This is more client-centered than simply indicating that she didn't follow our process. This is more client-centered than simply telling her she needs to go elsewhere, and use a different number or location. When a client arrives at any location, if any staff member at that community office or clinic is able to do an intake, such as the main telephone receptionist/intake worker would normally do, then that is what he should do. If a client calls the wrong number within the program, the person answering it should either complete the intake (if able to), or transfer the call directly to the intake staff, so the client still gets the intake done during the one phone call. Yes, these flexible approaches are inconvenient. No, it may not be the way we designed the process to work. Remember, though, that those things don't matter because *it's not about us*. It's about the client.

Actions for system managers and leaders:

Enable all staff at all locations to be able to welcome someone into the service, and at least do the basics of the administrative component to get an appointment booked for that client. Discourage staff from merely giving such a client a phone number, if she is there with the staff person anyway because of having dropped in. Empower staff to happily help engage the client into the service right there on the spot.

Actions for clients, supporters, and advocates:

1.   If your area has a single phone number or access point, try to use that if you can.

2.   If you cannot use that single access method, and the system has no flexibility to help you in another way, contact the program manager to explain what you need and why.

No Referral Needed

Many mental health programs have historically required clients to be referred to them by a physician. Most addiction programs have not had this practice, as people have generally been able to contact an addiction program directly and request service. This is often called a self-referral. The practice in mental health programs of requiring a referral from a doctor still exists today in some areas of Nova Scotia. In some cases, they have softened the language and refer to it as being "preferred" or "encouraged". Regardless of such language, it is still identified by the program as a relevant and important step in the process. Let's take a look at this approach, consider the advantages and disadvantages, and specifically analyze it from a client-centered perspective.

This approach fits within a traditional, medical-services model, in which patients cannot get access to a medical specialist (e.g., cardiologist, oncologist) without the need for such a specialty to first be identified by a general practitioner (i.e., family doctor). In other words, in a medical model, a doctor's referral is needed in order to see a specialist. Of course, this is often an appropriate step in medicine because it helps to maintain a structured system. It ensures that people only move on to the highest-trained specialists (i.e., professionals who are more scarce and more expensive in the system) if it is medically necessary. Otherwise, many of the symptoms being treated by family physicians might be taken directly to a specialist based solely on the concerns of the patient. Such situations would not take into account the very broad scope of services that can be provided by family physicians.

From an administrative and financial perspective, a structured system like this is efficient. It applies its human resources and its dollars according to the best fit with the presenting needs. From a client-centered perspective, such a structured model also makes sense to the extent that it ensures a proper match between the type and level of service and the type and level of need. Patients in a medical system should be neither under-treated nor over-treated.

There is, however, a major flaw in applying this specific medical process to the mental health and addiction system. The error is the inherent assumption that all the clients' needs are medical in nature. It assumes that there is a need for psychiatric intervention, and, therefore, must be cleared through a general practitioner first to ensure a legitimate need for medical specialist intervention. In other words, it assumes or implies that all clients need, or could benefit from, a psychiatrist (medical specialist), and therefore need a referral from a doctor. These assumptions and implications fit perfectly with the traditional medical and acute-care system, but they are misplaced in this context.

If we are looking to validate, or maintain, the traditional, medical/psychiatric paradigm for our mental health system, then a requirement for referral from a physician is completely appropriate. However, if we recognize the value of a tiered model to address all levels of need in a population appropriately, such an approach is a problem. If we want to move to a client-centered system in which all possible clients of this public program have access to the *appropriate* type and level of service for their own needs, then this approach is seriously flawed. It is a problem because only a minority of people require psychiatric/medical intervention to maintain or regain their mental health.

If the majority of potential and current clients do not require a psychiatrist, then that majority should also not require a physician referral. In fact, it should not even be "preferred" or encouraged. This is simply adding an additional, unnecessary inconvenience to the client's already difficult challenges. While it does serve the administrative need of placing physicians in the role of gatekeeper, and thereby reducing the perceived demand on the mental health and addiction system, it is not client-centered.

This required or preferred physician-referral process may also cause people to receive less than adequate care because of a mismatch of skills and client needs. Psychiatrists are medical doctors. Their primary education and training is in providing assessment and diagnosis of mental illness from a medical perspective, and then providing treatment, also from that medical perspective. Much of their work is neurology-based. The extent to which they develop skills in non-biomedical psychotherapy, or even less-intensive methods, like supportive counselling or life skills training, is very diverse. It depends on where they trained, what their individual level of interest was, and even their personalities and natural tendencies toward compassion, empathy, and strong interpersonal communication. Some have the skills to provide those less-intensive counselling services needed by many people, and some have skill sets that are limited to the medical types of interventions. It is entirely contingent on individual difference because that lower-end, less-intensive, earlier-intervention work is not a standard or fundamental part of the training. I know psychiatrists with whom I would trust my family for any level of support, and I have known psychiatrists who were brilliant specialists with no interpersonal skills or compassion.

There is an assumption in the current psychiatric, pathology-oriented paradigm that, as one moves up the professional hierarchy, there is a *cumulative* collection of skills. In other words, we assume that a counsellor can do counselling and life skills work only, but a therapist or clinical psychologist can do psychotherapy *as well as* the less-intensive counselling and life skills work, and that a psychiatrist can do the medical work *as well as* all those things that can be done by the psychologists, social workers, therapists and counsellors. This is an invalid assumption. In fact, it may be argued that the more-elevated a position one occupies in such an implied hierarchy, the narrower and more-specialized – and not the more-generalized – the skill set is.

If we have a system that encourages people to get a medical referral, or a system that channels all such referrals to a psychiatrist, we may be failing to provide appropriate or sufficient care to many clients by not matching the right skill set to their needs. Stories of people who feel their mental health issues are over-medicalized are not rare. We need to ensure that clients are channelled to the right kind of care, with people appropriately trained to provide it. We need to bust the myth that higher levels of specialized education mean a person has also accumulated the diversity of skills needed for the very distinct less-intensive types of interventions and supports that many need. These are *different* skill sets, with neither being more nor less important or necessary.

A client-centered public system that strives to serve *all* of its clients, not just those who are ill, requires all of these separate skill sets, and no single profession has them all. I even remember the days when it was assumed that any social worker or therapist could take on the role of a health promotion and prevention position in an addiction program. This seriously flawed thinking led to decades of wasted public dollars using completely ineffective prevention methods.

This assumed need for a medical referral is another reflection of the historical tendency to want to guard the castle and prevent people from getting in if they are not sick enough. A client-centered system intentionally and decisively removes steps that are pointless, in order for the client to receive the appropriate help. Therefore, unless there is a *medical* need for a person to see a doctor before coming to a mental health and addiction service, then he should not be sent there to jump through that unnecessary hoop. Also, unless there is a psychiatric (medical) reason for someone to see a psychiatrist, as opposed to having a psychological or psychosocial need, then he should not be sent to such a medical specialist.

It should also be fairly obvious how this contributes to increased wait times for clients. Suppose your sister is not feeling psychologically well, and calls her local mental health and addiction service to try to arrange to speak with someone. She is told either that it is preferred or required that she go to her doctor first to get a referral. First of all, she may perceive this as a form of rejection or lack of support or trust in her self-awareness, which can exacerbate the negative feelings that sent her there. Nonetheless, she hangs up and phones her family physician (if she has one) to seek an appointment. If she happens to have a physician who is running an advanced-access booking system, she may get a same-day appointment. However, given that such an approach is still not the norm in family medicine, she may be looking at waiting several weeks for that appointment. Meanwhile, her symptoms worsen. This is partly due to the simple passage of time, and partly due to the stress involved in waiting.

So, a few weeks have gone by and your sister arrives at the appointment with her doctor. When she meets with the physician and explains what is going on, and that she was told she needed a referral in order to see a therapist, the doctor really only has two main options. He can identify her as suffering from an anxiety or depression problem simply based on that conversation, and prescribe medication to address it. This can sometimes be less than ideal because medication may not be the appropriate or necessary solution for this particular client. The second option the doctor has is to make the referral to the mental health and addiction system. If he does that, it is based primarily on the client's self-report of need for that service. The doctor may also know things from her history that support her request, but if he has not noticed these issues in the past then this referral is still based solely on her self-reported need. It is based on the *same* information she already provided to the mental health and addiction system when she called. She said that's what she needed, she identified why (e.g., feeling sad, feeling anxious) and the doctor simply believes her and makes the referral to the mental health and addiction program, but not specifically to a psychiatrist because medical need is not indicated.

First, I would say kudos to the physician. Listening to the client's own self-identified needs and wishes and simply referring based on trust that the client knows herself is a client-centered approach. On the other hand, if a doctor used the first option of simply giving a prescription, client-centeredness was certainly questionable because she had asked for a referral to access counselling/therapy. She did not ask for medical intervention. If she had just come to the doctor saying "Here's what I'm feeling. How can you help?", that would be different because she is asking him to use his judgement about what she needs. In such a case, a prescription is not necessarily violating her sense of her own needs. It is, in fact, likely giving her what she has asked for.

So, let's follow the story a bit further. Suppose the doctor has done the most client-centered thing by making the referral as requested. The client now begins the process of waiting for the mental health and addiction appointment. In Nova Scotia, that wait could range from one to nine months, if not deemed to be an urgent or emergent case. What we have really done in such a case is take an already-lengthy wait time for mental health and addictions and added the primary care physician wait time to it. We are causing harm to our clients by adding in additional steps. This might be acceptable if those steps were necessary or productive. However, in this case, they are not.

If someone wants her physician's help, she can go ask for it and get it. But, if she wants access to a mental health and addiction service provider, that is different. Being redirected to her doctor so the doctor can simply fill out a paper or make a phone call just to legitimize her request is inefficient for the client, harmful to the progression of her symptoms, and may even be perceived as a sign of mistrust. All the doctor is verifying is that she says she has a certain kind of problem.

If this were your sister, how would you want this part of the system to work? That's easy. She knows if she needs to talk with somebody about her depression. She doesn't need a doctor to agree or to validate that self-awareness. She knows if she wants or needs to learn how to manage anxiety better. She does not need a physician to verify it just so she meets the inclusion criteria for our mental health and addiction system.

Consider this process from the broader perspective of efficiency in the health care system. In many areas, there are shortages of family physicians, and access is not always what we would like it to be. Yet, the mental health component of the system often forces those doctors and nurse practitioners to clog up their valuable appointments and increase wait times for their patients by having them go through an unnecessary rubber-stamping process.

Sure, these appointments are billable, so the physician is compensated. Sometimes, these appointments will be three or four minutes long and just a simple formality. At other times, they will be difficult for the physician, as the client will take up a significant amount of unplanned time. In either case, potentially-available physician appointments are lost, so clients who need to see their doctor directly for a medical need are waiting longer. Our primary care system simply cannot continue to be used as a gatekeeper for our mental health and addiction programs. If our mental health and addiction leaders do not think as part of a whole health care system, our programs will continue to cause these problems.

Please don't misunderstand. Family practitioners have a very significant role to play for those who come to them seeking help. Many of them have the skills and training to be able to listen and counsel, and, in some cases, medication will be an appropriate treatment. However, such a step should only be taken if it is the client's choice, and if there is an indication that medical issues underlie the mental health concern. Otherwise, our system disrespects the client's' time and right to self-determination, as well as directly causing further inefficiency in a stressed health care system.

Public mental health and addiction programs do not need a gatekeeper, or a moat around the castle. They also do not need to mistrust or question the legitimacy of a client's self-reported need, and delegate a validation process to doctors. They are meant to serve the public and, hence, need to be open and accessible to *all*. As described throughout this book, they are not meant to only serve those with a medical need. They have an obligation to serve all taxpayers at all levels of health and illness. Therefore, people without a medical/psychiatric need should be able to gain access without needing to jump through a medical hoop.

Actions for system managers and leaders:

Eliminate all requirements, encouragement, and even suggestions that clients see their doctor for a referral before coming into your mental health and addiction program. It is unnecessary, harmful to the client, and bad for the health care system.

Actions for clients, supporters, and advocates:

Find out if your local mental health and addiction program wants clients to get a referral from a doctor in order to get in. If it does, advocate for that to be eliminated, because it is bad for the clients and costs the health care system too much money and increased wait times in doctors' offices.

People Should Talk to a Human Being When They Call.

If the client were your father, how would you want the system to treat him when he first gets up the courage to call for help? If you are like most people, you would likely want someone to answer the phone. You would want to hear a person, not a recorded voice. You would not want a complicated series of automated options and buttons to push. People want to be treated with the respect of being responded to by another human being, as opposed to electronic response technology. That would reflect a client-centered approach.

We build *menu trees* into our phone systems regularly, in which you listen to recorded options and press numbers to try to get what you want or need. We often hear people argue that this is to simplify the phone call for the client, so he is directed to the place or person he is trying to reach. If it weren't for our propensity for rationalization, we administrators wouldn't be able to continue believing such falsehoods. A client is able to be connected to the right place far more effectively and efficiently (for the client) by another person than by an automated system. Who among us has not had the frustration of none of the recorded options sounding like what we need, but not being able to ask questions to clarify which is the right one?

Obviously, an automated phone system can save money by reducing the number of staff needed to answer telephones. Equally obvious is the fact that the health system in Canada is under significant financial pressure. These factors lead us to look for efficiencies and cheaper ways of doing things, such as using automated phone systems. If that is the case, and we choose to design such a system, then at least we should be forthright and aware of the fact that we are determining fiscal restraint to be a *higher priority* than providing a client-centered service. The money comes *prior to* the client in this case, which makes it system-centered. If this is the case, let's just acknowledge that fact and not spin it as better for the client.

Let's assume that a program administrator believes this to be a necessary sacrifice of client-centered principles because of the financial realities. That certainly is a valid consideration, but the population served by mental health and addiction programs will be disproportionately disadvantaged compared with the general population accessing other services. In other words, setting up an automated phone system with recorded voices and buttons to push is more harmful for potential clients of a mental health and addiction program than it would be for clients of another kind of health service. The experience of anxiety, depression, social isolation, paranoia, insecurity, trauma, rejection, etc., that these clients live every day increases their need for warmth, compassion, and empathy in order to develop a sense of trust and safety. Without that comfort level, they will be less likely to engage with the service they need.

A recorded voice doesn't provide that. Clients often experience it as cold, impersonal, and another sign that they are not important or valuable enough as individuals to deserve for their calls to be answered by a person. The way clients are received and welcomed should fit their experiences and needs, and facilitate their getting the care they require. We would never consider putting an orthopedic clinic for people with knee and hip problems on the second floor of a building with no elevator. Requiring them to use stairs would be ridiculous because of the *specific* nature of their illness. For a different client population, stairs may not be a problem. Establishing anything short of a warm and empathic human voice on the end of the phone line when someone calls a mental health and addiction program is equally inappropriate. It is a direct barrier to access, as much as stairs for people seeking knee replacement, because it inadvertently puts an obstacle in front of their *specific* area of illness. Therefore, even if health care managers believe it is a justifiable sacrifice of client-centered principles to put finances first with the use of automated phone systems, such a sacrifice must not apply to mental health and addiction programs and their clients because of the unique nature of the empathic care they need.

Actions for system managers and leaders:

Eliminate automated answering services and recorded menu trees, and replace them with people answering the phone.

Actions for clients, supporters, and advocates:

If your local system does not have real people answering the main telephone line, contact the program management and tell them it is better for the clients if they switch to people.

People Should Talk to a Genuinely
Nice Person When They Call

As discussed, there are several ways to give potential clients a choice of options and ensure they are connected to the right people. Only one of those is capable of friendliness, warmth, comfort, empathy, and compassion. That is what distinguishes a real person from a machine, and is why most people prefer to hear a nice person on the other end of the phone. Not surprisingly, people dealing with mental health challenges tend to value, if not require, empathy and compassion. Clients are comforted by a warm and friendly voice and conversation on the end of the line when they have just made what might be the scariest or most embarrassing phone call of their lives. The position of receptionist in many organizations is sometimes jokingly, but affectionately, referred to as the 'director of first impressions'. That is the most important function of the people answering the phone or greeting clients when they make contact or arrive for an appointment. This person has to be passionate about making the client feel valued, important, respected, safe, and comfortable. A recorded voice on a phone, or a live but insincere person, can't do any of those things, and may in fact undermine and prevent clients from experiencing those very important feelings.

Any competent and reasonably organized employee can learn the procedural parts of that important job. They can learn to gather and enter information into software, while questioning a client on the phone or registering her at the desk upon arrival. This is in no way to suggest it is an easy job to do reception and intake work. It is to suggest, however, that there is a distinction between technical skills that can be taught/learned and personal qualities and skills that cannot. While people can learn to ask questions and record answers into client information software, they can't learn to have a pleasant, warm, and welcoming personality. Personality, by definition, is the collection of traits that make us distinct from one another. The stability of such traits is what makes it different from variable constructs such as moods. Moods change, while personality traits generally do not. People who are not naturally and consistently pleasant and compassionate can try to fake it, but genuineness and phoniness are two things we all seem well-equipped to detect. Clients will know.

Can you recall entering a business, a health clinic, or maybe even a restaurant, and being greeted by someone who said the right, friendly words, and displayed a smile, but clearly was just playing a role and didn't really care? Can you recall the opposite, when you sensed that a genuinely pleasant and friendly personality was behind that smile? Of course. So, to have the *right* person answer the main telephone line in a mental health and addiction program, people must be hired according to personality, and then trained to develop the technical and procedural skills. Hire for warmth, optimism, patience, empathy, and trait-based friendliness. That is what the client population in a mental health and addiction program specifically needs because of the nature of their concerns or illnesses. That would be a client-centered approach to staffing because the hiring would be based entirely on what best fits the needs of these specific clients, not on the efficiency, technical, or data-related needs of our programs. *It's not about us.* It's about the client.

Actions for system managers and leaders:

For all telephone or office reception and intake positions, hire based on genuineness, warmth, friendliness, and the natural tendency to actually demonstrate empathy, compassion, positivity, and optimism. Then train them on the technical skills.

Actions for clients, supporters, and advocates:

If your local program has someone answering the phone, or greeting clients in a reception area, who is not genuinely nice to people, tell the program manager, so she can look into the situation and fix it.

CHAPTER 7

HELPING CLIENTS GET INTO THE SYSTEM CONVENIENTLY

In the previous chapter, we discussed making the system efficient, appropriate, and welcoming for clients as they initiate contact for the purpose of receiving service. Now, let's assume we have fixed that part of the process so it is designed to be about the client. Furthermore, let's assume we have a client on the phone in a comfortable conversation, looking to get an appointment booked. How will it turn out? Will he get an appointment booked? Will it be soon? Will it be convenient for his life schedule? The answer to such questions is determined by the extent to which client access and availability of appointments is treated as the *priority*. In other words, does that factor come first before other operational needs? Does it come *prior* to other things in practice, not just in words or statements of principle?

What would a client-centered system look like in this part of the process? If the client were your son, how would you want it to work? Well, presumably, you would want a system that constantly works to remove barriers that get in the way of access. Let's look at how to do that within a client-centered paradigm.

Eliminate Barriers to Convenient and Timely Access

I will start by saying **let's NOT start by saying** *we need more money and staff*. While that may sometimes be the case, often it is not. It is

114

an assumption. It is an easy go-to solution because it requires far less work than transforming the system. Unfortunately, it has the appeal of being a simple, immediate, and prevailing excuse for *not* transforming the system. One easy way to avoid having to apply the creativity and innovation of leadership, and then having to maneuver the very complicated and often unpopular work of change management, is to identify a significant external barrier to progress, over which we have no control. Not enough money, staff, or clinical services certainly fit that bill.

This default approach prevents us not only from doing the hard work, but also from having to learn or develop the skills of leadership if we don't have them already. Taking this a step further, many people prefer to have that type of defensive argument because it keeps them from failing. The blame for any mistakes or problems or ongoing criticisms of the system never falls to those running the services. As long as the overall problem is perceived to be really about those big factors that governments control, blame can always be deflected to them, and the system leaders never feel like, or are perceived as, failing to do their job. "We are doing the best we can with what we have," becomes the common refrain.

In order to make such a statement about needing more money and staff, and be certain that we are correct, we would need to have assurance that all of the resources we currently have are being used to their full capacity and in accordance with a full understanding of the client being *the priority*. There's the catch. Only a truly client-centered approach will ensure the maximization of capacity within the program. Once a system has been transformed in this way, and we can be reasonably sure that money and staff time are not being used to serve administrative, professional, political, or personal needs of the system and the people working within it, we are in a different place. It may then be valid for leadership to say that any remaining gap needs to be addressed through additional resources. Until that time, we need to stop taking the easy way out, and start taking responsibility (credit and blame) for our actions or inactions toward fundamental change. Until that time, the money argument is merely hypothetical.

We must eliminate barriers to access. We must find efficiencies for clients, not for the system, in our public mental health and addiction services. We must recognize that every decision we make about past, present, and future ways of doing things is a decision about prioritization, and where the client fits in this concept of *relative* importance. The rest of this chapter and the next examine some of the common barriers to access, and suggest how this would be handled if we shifted from the current, expert-driven, psychiatric paradigm to one that is client-centered.

Actions for system managers and leaders:

Complete the suggested transformations in this book (plus many others that you similarly may identify) before claiming to need more money or staff.

Actions for clients, supporters, and advocates:

If money is claimed as the barrier in your local area, ask about the transformations described here to see if they have already been completed. If you can see that they have, then help advocate for more money or identify additional funding sources. If not, advocate first for these client-centered changes.

Barrier – No Appointments That Fit Clients' Schedules and Life Pressures.

As briefly described earlier, most mental health and addiction programs, certainly in Nova Scotia, have historically provided their outpatient services Monday to Friday during daytime hours only. This is by nature a system-centric model. It is designed around program efficiency, easy staff scheduling, and preferred work hours of staff in the organization. In other words, it is designed around the needs of the program and the people working in it. While this was noted in an earlier chapter, a few more relevant and specific points are needed here in the context of barriers.

What would a client-centered approach look like? If the client were your brother, how would you want it to work? To the greatest extent possible, the system needs to provide a diversity of options to allow the scheduling of an appointment that fits each client's life. If it is actually client-centered, then the schedule would allow people to get an appointment during evenings, weekends, early mornings before work, etc.

Why is this important? You may think this is an issue of convenience for the client and, in part, you would be right. The job of a public program is to make their services as accessible and convenient as possible for the taxpayers who fund them. However, there are also noteworthy ethical considerations regarding our obligation to cause no harm. The clients our programs are supposed to serve are struggling with various aspects of their day-to-day lives, trying to cope with stressors, and attempting to manage the overwhelming feelings that can arise when experiencing early or later symptoms of mental illness. They do not need our programs to give them more duress and pain. They do not need the mental health and addiction service to cause yet another inconvenience, pressure, scheduling conflict, or logistical complication they must try to handle.

With the traditional limitations on hours of operation, programs do cause more pressure by making clients fit into a narrow scope of appointment times that may not align with their already-busy and complicated lives. In other words, the program is potentially causing further exacerbation of the very health issues it is supposed to help mitigate. Ever been in such a situation? Have you needed to get an appointment for some kind of service (e.g., health care, auto repair, banking), but found the scheduling limits made it stressful because they did not fit your life and obligations? Is that the unpleasant experience you would want for your brother if he needed some type of mental health care appointment? I doubt it. From a client perspective, that is a problem. From an organizational ethics perspective, it is an even-more-serious problem because of the risk of further harming a person's well-being.

The second area of ethical concern with traditional weekday hours is the financial harm it can cause to clients. Any client who has a daytime job that does not include paid sick-time for health care appointments will need to take time off work to attend. If lucky, depending on the way the employer does the scheduling, that might mean just a loss of an hour or two. If unlucky, it could mean the loss of a shift and a full day's wages. It is also likely in these situations that this is a low-paying job, not a stable higher-paying career, as the latter usually allows for such time off and the former does not.

Causing a loss of income in this way for clients is simply unacceptable. Income is a determinant of health. In health care, we use this language all the time. We say we need to work on the determinants of health, but yet we allow systems to be designed that cause harm with regard to the most important and influential global determinant of health – money. If the client were your brother, how would you want it to work? Likely, you would want to have appointments that allow more diverse options in terms of days of the week and times of the day, so he would not need to choose between income to feed his family and receiving mental health care for himself (which may also be related to the same financial stress).

People in the system will cite barriers to being able to move in this direction. For example, they will talk about difficulties making the change in a unionized environment because it may cause the unions to file grievances about scheduling or to look for more money in the form of a premium for evening or weekend work. Depending on the way job descriptions have been written and what the established norms are for an estoppel argument, there may be some negotiation needed. But, generally speaking, unless there have ever been commitments to only weekday and daytime hours, or unless job descriptions provide that guarantee, this is not as complicated as some would lead us to believe. It is a great example of an argument that often stops managers from making system changes, even when not valid. Besides that, some unions and some union representatives (not all) are willing to support such client-centered changes.

Even in unionized situations in which the current, negotiated agreement doesn't allow for such scheduling, that does not mean we can't proceed. It means we need to negotiate a change to that agreement. If a road we are driving on is blocked, we don't just stop and live there in our car forever, or turn around and go home... we take another, perhaps less convenient, route and keep moving toward our intended destination. So, negotiate. Maybe it will cost more money if the union does not share our principles about client-centeredness. That would be unfortunate, but would just bring us back to deciding between money and client well-being. It is still possible to do it, but it will require a client-centered decision about *priority.* Either way, someone has to spend or lose money that they don't have. Either the program overspends, or the client loses wages that are needed for rent or food. If we are client-centered, that doesn't seem like a complicated decision.

The system needs to be designed around providing appointments that fit the clients' lives, not the lives of the staff or management, and not the unions' preferences. In a client-centered paradigm, all those parties would be working collaboratively and in accordance with the same principle. Client-centered means client-centered, and all those parties need to understand and internalize the idea that *it's not about us.* It is about the client.

Actions for system managers and leaders:

Build a schedule that provides appointments during days, evenings, early mornings, weekends, to the greatest extent possible, and make sure all clients are made fully aware of those options so they can choose what works for them.

Actions for clients, supporters, and advocates:

Request appointments that fit your life. If they are not available, let the management and leadership of the program know that it is important to make that change. You never know... there may be managers or staff who naively believe nobody wants these other times available, just because nobody ever asked.

Barrier – Services are not Where Clients Need Them to Be

All the arguments made in the previous section apply in principle to the issue of geography and location of services. The often-cited real-estate mantra "location, location, location" is extremely relevant to a client-centered paradigm. Clients cannot access services if they cannot get to where they are located.

In large metropolitan areas, which may have effective public transportation, part of this issue may be reduced for some people. In rural areas, that is clearly not the case. Travelling to centralized offices far from their own communities is often very difficult and expensive, if not *impossible*, for clients. In addition, regardless of urban or rural locations, and regardless of methods of transportation available, the farther a service is from where a person lives or works, the bigger the disruption to his day because of travel time. That simply adds to the life pressures and potential loss of income described in the previous section. Even in urban areas, services need to be decentralized if we want them to be client-centered. The idea of having services all clustered in one location, requiring that clients go to them, is an outdated model that is based on institutional, medical-model thinking. It fits well with intensive inpatient services, but, unfortunately, has also been generalized and applied to all outpatient work over recent decades. That is one of the reasons why mental health and addiction programs operated by and within a hospital will very often fail to develop client-centered outpatient services, and will often receive much public criticism about access.

What does a client-centered service look like in terms of geography? It is decentralized, rather than being entirely based in a main location to which all clients are expected to travel. Quite literally, the more community-based locations there are, the more client-centered the service is. Outpatient work should be based in as many community locations as possible. This is a key reason why integration of services into primary care clinics and schools is so beneficial. It is bringing the help to where people already are. It simplifies their lives, provides them with choice, and saves them time, stress, and money. It reduces the harm that our traditional, centralized, institutional, and medical-model systems cause.

Having implemented various approaches to this decentralization of services several times, in many geographic areas, and in several kinds of health services, I can tell you that the idea regularly elicits a case of the *'yeah buts'*. Start suggesting moving staff out of a central location and into doctor's offices, schools, or new satellite clinics, and many people will start to say things like *"Yeah, but we need all our staff here to keep up with the demand."* or *"Yeah, but that will leave the rest of us with more work here than we can handle."* The *yeah buts* will drag any program into maintaining the *status quo* faster than lightening. It will keep a program system-centered against all rational or principle-based arguments. It casts unreasonable doubt on the feasibility of any option.

In reality, putting the *yeah buts* aside, there are a few predictable outcomes of this decentralizing. First of all, the location where the clients are served will shift. Prospectively speaking, new clients who would normally have booked appointments at the main central office, will now book them at a more-convenient location, thereby reducing demand on the central office at the same time staffing is reduced there. Essentially, some of the demand simply shifts so it follows the staff because the clients will gravitate toward the most convenient location (one of the very reasons we need to do it). Second, because of increased convenience, people will start to access services earlier in their distress, symptoms, or illness – because they can.

The impact of this approach is twofold. It actually does mean a potential increase in numbers of clients served. However, it also means briefer and more effective work because it represents earlier intervention than the system typically provides. This is described in more detail in a previous discussion on early intervention. This second outcome (more people coming for help, but earlier) is yet another of the reasons we *need* to move in this direction intentionally.

Actions for system managers and leaders:

Decentralize. Disperse your *existing* staff to as many convenient community locations as possible. Put them in schools, primary care clinics, or community centers.

> **Actions for clients, supporters, and advocates:**
>
> Suggest and advocate for services to be moved into your local area. Explain to the management or the elected officials how the geographic unavailability negatively affects you. Don't assume they understand the real harm in your life caused by centralized services. Many will not have ever considered this impact.

Reducing Unexpected Disruptions to Service

A quote was recently posted online and attributed to former boxing champion Mike Tyson as follows: "Everyone has a plan... until they get punched in the face." From a system perspective, what this means is you can design and implement everything discussed in this book, and still have things disrupt or get in the way of client service. Staff members get sick or are injured, have personal emergencies or family crises, and basically unwanted and unpredicted things happens. These kinds of events, along with weather-related disruptions, can cause gaps in service. This can happen by virtue of one, many, or even all clinicians not being present, services being shut down, or clients being unable to make it in for their appointments. While we clearly don't have any control over these events taking place, we do have some ability to be intentional and client-centered in the way we respond to them.

Unexpected Staff Absences

Suppose a clinician notifies the clinic that he is going to be unexpectedly absent due to illness or some other such issue. Consider the features of this situation. We have a clinician who won't be present and clients who are booked for that clinician. Often, and perhaps instinctively, programs go into cancellation mode to make sure all those clients are notified and rescheduled if possible. This is the normal approach in many health care services, as it is the standard in a medical paradigm. However, in doing this, we have failed to look at the rest of the circumstances, and have failed to look at this from a client-centered perspective.

If we break the situation down a little further, we can easily identify that some of the clients who are booked may be well established and engaged in a healthy therapeutic relationship with that absent clinician. This limits our ability to meet that client's needs today with another clinician, in the way they would have been addressed in the planned session. But, it does not prevent us from helping that client to manage any kind of crisis he might be experiencing.

In these kinds of situations, clients are rarely asked what they would prefer. We just proceed to call and reschedule with the same clinician, probably several weeks or months away. What if we were to ask clients about their preferences? Is it possible that, once in a while, we would discover a client who has been anxiously awaiting the appointment because of some challenging things going on in her life? If so, is it possible that she may choose to see some other therapist at the originally-scheduled time, if there is one available, simply for those more-urgent issues? A client-centered approach to this situation would lead us to see this as a good option. In any cases in which a clinician has non-clinical things scheduled during that particular day, we need to ask ourselves which of these items is the *priority*. Is it making sure that the case notes get done at that time, or that a clinician does not have to miss some or all of a meeting? From a client-centered perspective, the answer is *no*. If the client is at the *center*, and if the client is the *priority*, that means the needs of that client at that time come *prior to* the other responsibilities of the staff in the program. *It's not about us.*

So, a manager could reassign whomever is not scheduled for a clinical session, and have him help his absent colleague's client to manage her immediate challenge or crisis. It may just save a life. In other words, rather than habitually just cancelling the clients of the clinician who perhaps called in sick, we could ask the client if she wants to be seen by someone else (if there is some clinician time available, i.e., not scheduled for a clinical appointment with another client at that time).

When someone is out unexpectedly, there will also be the possibility that one or more of the clients who were supposed to be seen that day are new clients. If that is the case, then any clinician who is free (i.e., not booked with a client at that time) could see that new client. He is not yet attached to any therapist, has no rapport or therapeutic relationship established, and so can easily be reassigned at the last minute.

Once again, if we were to ask staff working in the traditional paradigm if this was possible or ideal, we may get concerns related to their having enough work to do, needing time to do paperwork, needing a break once in a while from the intensive clinical work, or perhaps meetings being important. It cannot be stated assertively enough that those things are very important. But, this isn't about whether or not such things are important. This is about the concept of *priority*.

In a situation with competing pressures, no matter what we do we will end up making a decision about which factor is *more or most* important. If we let things operate the way we currently do, and simply reschedule that client, we **have made a decision by default** that one or more of those reasons possibly identified by staff above is, in fact, *a higher priority than* this new client to whom we have committed.

It is my observation that many of the people running our programs would never concede this point. They would never agree that in these situations they are actually making a choice to favor administrative tasks over client needs, and on some level they are probably right. The concept of a choice or a decision implies some level of consciousness and intentionality, which is not always there in these cases. Many of these day-to-day, system decisions are more like automated or habituated responses based on historical ways of doing things. They are determined by the culture into which each staff person, manager, leader is assimilated when they join the program. They adapt to, and become part of, the system.

This is not much different from one of the common public observations about politics. Generally, good, principled people run for office in democratic societies. Regardless of that fact, once they are inside government, in a partisan system, the re-election machine takes over. All those good people then do their best to make a difference, *within the constraints of the way things work*. Assimilation into a culture with its own way of making decisions, and its own corporate/political attitudes, norms, and expectations, is a very powerful and usually invisible process. Its primary function, as suggested by systems theory, is to maintain homeostasis. In other words, the job of a system and its culture, is to protect that system from changing. That is why most people don't even realize they have been assimilated.

Any Star Trek fans reading this may have already had a vision of the Borg. What I am talking about is not that different, except that, in this case, resistance is *not* futile. It can be changed. The key point here is that our leaders in the mental health and addiction programs need to stop allowing the system to keep functioning the same way. They need to change processes *intentionally* – like how we respond to unexpected staff absences. We should not and cannot just uncritically accept the historical norm, and assume that because we are good people our program is therefore client-centered. Practices must change to allow some of those clients to be seen the same day even if their clinician is unexpectedly absent, recognizing that the non-clinical activities of the other clinicians are *a lower priority.*

Actions for system managers and leaders:

When responding to an unplanned clinician absence, ask that your intake team:

1. Determine which clinicians may have non-clinical time available that day, and when.

2. Ask the *established* clients of the absent clinician if they want or need to see a different person that day, or to be rescheduled with their usual clinician for a later date. This leaves the client with choice and self-determination.

3. For any *new* client, unless there is a clinical reason why he needs to see that specific absent clinician, reassign him to another clinician who can see him at the planned appointment time. This ensures no additional waiting, planning, disruption to employment, cost, etc., to the client, as the program is bending and adapting in order to keep its commitment to have a therapist see him that day.

Actions for clients, supporters, and advocates:

If you receive a cancellation or rescheduling call, and you need support that day, ask if you can see someone else. In a traditional and rigid program, the answer may be no, and you may be told there is nobody available. But, merely asking the question might start people thinking about this option. Additionally, you could advocate with the management of your local program for this kind of approach to be adopted in order to reduce inconvenience and disruption to clients' already-established plans and expectations.

Weather-Related Disruptions

In Canada, especially in winter, there are days when bad weather causes significant disruption to staff members' ability to get to work, and the program's ability to continue to offer service. Some of these situations precisely fit the previous discussion. If an individual clinician is unable to make it to work because of weather, this is a similar circumstance to illness or another personal situation, except for the fact the clinician may still be able to do work at home. If we take a client-centered approach to this kind of situation, the important question is whether or not there is still a way to deliver service to at least some of the scheduled clients, despite the fact that staff members or clients may be unable to travel to the office because of weather or road conditions.

This depends on the nature of the client's issues and how well-established the clinical relationship is. If the clinical relationship and the client's health are reasonably stable, it may be possible to proceed with a telephone session. This is complicated, especially from a privacy perspective. But, *complicated* does not mean impossible or inappropriate. Presenting the option to the client would be the first reasonable step, and one that keeps the client in complete control and ensures that her needs are met. Some will choose not to do so because it is not the kind of communication they are comfortable having, or because there are other people at home who they don't want to have overhear their clinical conversation. Others, however, may not want to wait for several more weeks (or months depending on how long a program's wait times are) for the rescheduled appointment.

The client-centered approach would be to give him the choice. If he chooses to proceed with a phone session, then the privacy conditions must be established and understood. The client, of course, has the right to ensure that he is in a private room where no one else can hear, or can choose to have this conversation elsewhere in the house with other family members or friends present. It is his information, and it is never a privacy breach, under any circumstances, for a client to choose to share it. That is his choice completely, despite our tendency toward paternalistic attempts to protect him from his own decisions.

On the clinician's end, it is a different story. The clinician would need to ensure that she is in a location where no one else could learn of the client's identity or private health information. For many people, this would certainly be possible by being in a separate room not adjacent to where others are in the clinician's home. Protecting privacy on that end is the clinician's legal and ethical obligation and must be met. It is simple for a program, with advice from its privacy experts, to develop criteria that would need to be met to enable such sessions to happen.

Any time we engage in clinical sessions by telephone, we must also take precautions regarding boundaries and perceived relationships. It must be clear to the client that this is a scheduled, professional session and not a social call or a call between friends, even though it is happening at home. If that is not clearly understood, we run the risk of harm to the client and compromising clinical effectiveness through creating a real or perceived dual relationship. In addition, the clinician should have the technological capacity to block her own personal phone number when making the call to the client for the session. Sharing one's personal number also potentially leads to false impressions about the relationship, and could lead to further contact at home based on that perception.

We must do what is best for the client, and is best for the broader public we serve. If we have the ability to respond differently to unforeseen circumstances like weather, and thereby prevent a further increase in wait times, we must do so. It is the obligation of a public service to work creatively and innovatively to make options like this work.

Actions for system managers and leaders:

1. Develop criteria to clarify the privacy conditions that need to be met in order for clinical sessions to happen by phone from a clinician's home.

2. When weather causes a clinician to be unable to get to the office, but she is still able to work from home, place the continuation of the planned clinical session at the top of the priority list for her day, and ensure she gives the client the choice, and then meets all the privacy criteria before beginning a session.

Actions for clients, supporters, and advocates:

1. If given this option on the stormy day of a scheduled appointment, consider the benefit of not having to wait and reschedule, and then try the phone option if you are comfortable with it. Remember, if you start the phone call, and don't like it, you can simply end the conversation and reschedule your appointment. You are never trapped into anything like this simply by trying it.

2. If you or your loved one receive a cancellation call on a stormy day, and if you think a phone session would be better than rescheduling, ask for one even if it is not offered. The program may agree, but, if not, it's an opportunity to advocate for this client-centered option to be provided.

CHAPTER 8

HELPING CLIENTS GET INTO THE SYSTEM QUICKLY

Let's talk math. Begin looking at what all the clinicians' time is being used for, and add up the amount of it that is not spent directly supporting and treating clients. You may be shocked. In the following sections, we will explore ways to improve the timeliness of access, specifically through the elimination of some of the most-common, time-related barriers. These factors are all identified as barriers because they reduce the amount of clinical time available, and raise the key question of *priority* in the use of such time. Start with the basic idea that one hour spent by a therapist doing something other than therapy is one more hour added to the collective wait time for clients trying to get in. It is an appointment that is taken away and is unavailable for a client to use.

Barrier – Internal Meetings

It seems like just a meeting here and there, but it adds up to increased wait times when totalled. Let's assume that a program's clinical staff meet for two hours a week to review new client referrals. This is one of the historical methods of assigning clients that, thankfully, is disappearing in the field. Maybe the program has multiple sites, and there are some staff meetings at each of those locations. Let's suggest, minimally, that there is a total of just 20 staff in these meetings. That amounts to 40 hours per week of publicly-paid clinical time not being used to see clients. That is, on average, 30-40 clinical appointments every single week not available for people trying to get in for help. Simple math.

As we evolve, and old, meeting-based approaches to processes like case assignment are eliminated, the wait time can be instantly reduced by weeks simply through the cancellation of that one weekly meeting. As noted in an earlier chapter, there is no reason for such meetings in a public service because they are based on a process of individual staff selecting which clients they will or can accept. While normal and appropriate in private practice, it is not so in public service. If, individually, clinicians have no say in such a selection process, then the meeting is irrelevant.

Staff meetings for non-clinical purposes also occur on a regular basis in most programs. Clearly, there is a need for some such meetings, but the frequency and amount of time allotted should be contingent on the purpose of the meeting and whether a meeting is *really needed*, or just preferred, in order to meet those purposes.

For example, if the purpose of a staff meeting is simply to provide information to employees about policies, changes, directions, etc., such one-way communication can be done by email, group voice message, or other such approaches. If the purpose is to allow for necessary interaction, such as using a meeting to develop those policies, changes, and directions, then it must be determined how that can be achieved with as little clinical time used as possible. That might mean a very brief meeting for all staff and a smaller representative group doing the work (thereby reducing the overall number of clinical person-hours used). However, the development of policy and direction is more appropriately a management task. This does not imply a non-empowering or non-collaborative authoritarian style of management. It implies that the bulk of the time-consuming part of the work of such policy and program development should not be done by staff whom the public pays for therapy. It is not their primary skill set, it is not what they were trained or hired to do, and it is not client-centered to use that resource that way at the expense of clients who are waiting.

The appropriate approach is to find the balance that first achieves the right client-centered use of clinical time, while also providing as much opportunity for staff empowerment and staff input as possible. That may mean management getting input as often and efficiently as possible, so that the general directions that are then developed by management are already inclusive of the clinical staff perspective, without their putting in the time developing the details and the documents. This is easily done in an open-door management environment, in hallway chats, in targeted questions of specific staff between sessions. The point is that input can be gathered to ensure good program development, without taking clinical appointments away from clients and increasing the wait time. Consultation and inclusiveness of staff in program directions, policies, and management functions does not need to take the form of time-consuming meetings. It can often just be a dynamic management process of always gathering people's thoughts, beliefs, and ideas, and perpetually synthesizing them into collective input for program direction. A hundred, two-minute, intentional conversations can often be worth far more, and can more accurately reflect the views of staff, than one meeting all together for a couple hours. It is sometimes more effective at getting every person's views, especially those who generally will not speak in a group setting.

When meetings must include clinical staff, using telephone or video calls in place of face-to-face meetings is recommended, particularly if meetings would require clinicians travelling from multiple sites to a meeting. This allows a one-hour meeting to only take one hour, rather than one hour plus travel time. Also, setting the length of the meetings to the minimum needed, and no more, is another strategy for reducing negative impacts on client access. A wise mentor of mine has always said a meeting will take whatever amount of time you schedule for it. If you set it for an hour, it will take an hour, but if you set that same meeting for two hours, the content and discussion will expand to fill that time.

Many have written about producing efficiency in meetings through various methods that create brevity, like standing up instead of sitting, or creating a culture of quick, bullet-type exchanges as opposed to open narrative discussion. Also, as agendas are built, items that are merely information-sharing and can be done outside of meetings often find their way onto the agenda, nonetheless. That needs to be strictly managed, and that can only happen if the meeting is run by someone with the specific skill set of chairing and facilitating work meetings, not clinical discussions. The main point is that when staff meetings *are* required, the time allotted, the style of meeting, the frequency, the agenda items, and the way it is chaired, among other factors, should be designed and structured to *minimize* impact on clinical time available for appointments. In other words, it is important to keep the client as the priority as much as possible and manage that tightly.

For every meeting, for every agenda item, for every decision about who should attend, how long will it be, where or through what technology it will be held, here is the question that must repeatedly be asked – Is this a *more* important use of a clinician's time than a client getting an appointment sooner? Remember in a client-centered paradigm, there is no place for merely saying something is important. There is only room for saying if one thing is *more* or *less* important than another. In the context of this current discussion and the impact on wait times, for instance, we must ask if client access is less important than any particular meeting you are considering? More to the paradigm shift proposed in this book, if your daughter were the client, which would you consider more important, and how would you want this choice to be made?

Actions for system managers and leaders:

1. Critically challenge the assumptions about the relative importance of all kinds of staff meetings, in comparison with the increase in wait times that they **directly** cause.

2. Reduce the frequency, length, and number of people attending all such meetings to *first* improve access, and *second* allow for the minimum meeting time needed to run the program.

Barrier – External Meetings

One of the other things that takes clinicians away from seeing clients, and thereby diminishes the amount of program capacity and increases wait times, is staff involvement in outside meetings and events. The same math applies here as in all other cases. For every two hours that a clinician spends at any kind of community meeting, that is two hours of clinical appointment time no longer available for clients trying access services. That is two more hours added to the cumulative wait time.

Let's consider this specifically from a client-centered perspective. First, what are the competing priorities here that need to be appropriately *ranked* to ensure the client comes first? For example, when there is a community or interagency committee on which the mental health and addiction program should be represented, there are several questions to ask. Is it a clinical meeting? Will the discussions be about cases, clients, and clinical issues? Or, will it be about interagency partnerships, processes, collaborative initiatives, policies, or even politics?

The answers to these questions should determine the type of staff position that would represent the best fit and the best use of program resources. In this example, if it is not specifically a clinical meeting dealing with client issues, then the question becomes – 'Is attendance at this meeting a *more*-important use of publicly-funded, clinical staff hours than seeing clients?'. From a client-centered perspective, this would be an inappropriate prioritization. Those hours should go back into the bank of available time for seeing clients. If, on the other hand, the meeting was for the purpose of talking about certain clients, or specific approaches to clinically-collaborative work, then it would make sense for clinical representation to be present.

Clinical collaboration rightfully belongs high on the priority list because it has potential to improve effectiveness of the work with any particular client. However, it is still important for management of the program to protect the availability of clinical time vigilantly. If there is no good reason to have more than one clinical representative at the clinically-collaborative meeting, then that should not happen. If it is about an individual client, then the staff members directly involved with that client are the right ones. If it is about clinical processes not attached to a specific client, then one clinician, or someone from management with a clinical background, might be the right representative. Otherwise, the program is unnecessarily spending more hours from that bank of available client time.

Whether an external committee or meeting becomes an ongoing time commitment (e.g., monthly, quarterly) should be determined and reconsidered on a regular basis for its usefulness and for its relevance to the use of clinical staff. Many committees start off with one intention but end up having much more general, looser, often less-productive conversations as time goes on. Program management and staff must monitor that closely so they can pull back clinical time when it appears to be not well spent, when compared to using it for client access. Remember, everything is a question about *relative* importance, not just importance.

Regardless of how busy the managers and leaders of the program are, the use of their time for non-clinical meetings makes more sense. If we really mean it when we say the program is client-centered, we would not take away a client's access to a clinical session in order to have a therapist attend a meeting that is not clinically necessary. Both things *cannot* be the priority. One has to pick, and picking client-centered in this case will help fix the system.

Perhaps, we can think of it this way. Among all the kinds of positions in a public mental health and addiction program, the paid hours of those who directly serve clients are the ones that should be protected the most. If there is a need to take time from the schedules of people in the program to attend a meeting, management should be used first and client-service staff should be used last. That is just another example of prioritization.

Managers reading this are likely thinking this implies their time is not important, or implies that they even have time available. Neither is intended. I have spent my career on that treadmill. But, remember, this is not about what is important. It is about *priority*, and therefore about *ranking* and identifying all the things that are *less* important than the client and in this case his access and wait times. Protecting the direct-service hours for the client is the top priority here, above all others, including management time. That is, in fact, what the taxpayers fund those clinical hours for. And, for anyone in management, *it's not about us.*

Actions for system managers and leaders:

Only assign clinical staff to outside meetings if those meetings are specifically clinical in nature, and therefore actually **require** clinical participation. Even then, limit such participation to either those directly involved with the clients being discussed, or to a clinical representative, to reduce the number of overall clinical hours we add to the wait time.

Barrier – Workshops and Conferences

Every year, every month, practically every week, staff in mental health and addiction programs receive notices of presentations, webinars, workshops, and conferences. Individual staff read them, see them as interesting or useful for their own professional growth, and put in a request to management to attend. For some, this is a genuine attempt to become better at their jobs. For some, this is an opportunity to learn about something not directly related to their jobs but that is personally or professionally interesting, nonetheless. Then, there are those same small few who put in the request because it is an opportunity to get a day off work. Thankfully, that last group is tiny, but every workplace in the world has a couple of those folks.

First, it must be acknowledged that professional development has value. But, to address this situation from a client-centered perspective, we must first understand that the concept of *value* is on a continuum, and it is yet another *relative* term. Saying it is on a continuum simply means that our decision isn't just *whether or not* something has value.

Everything has value and falls somewhere along a line between a little and a lot.

Second, to say that the word value is a *relative* term again means that where something sits on the *value* continuum is determined by its relationship to something else. This makes it similar to the way this book has described the word priority. For purposes of this discussion, the value of something like staff educational opportunity is primarily contingent on its perceived usefulness in achieving a person's or organization's goals. For example, if a web-based learning opportunity came around that needed to be done outside of work hours, it would be perceived to have utility to those looking to improve their work and also to those looking to expand their own minds, but would not be perceived as useful by the person looking to get a day off. By the same logic, a mundane workshop during paid time would be useful to the work-avoidant group but not to the two categories of people who are interested in learning. Finally, a workshop about an essential, but not stimulating, work-related process would be useful to those looking to improve their job performance, and to those looking to get a day off, but not to those looking to stimulate their minds. The value of something like professional development is contingent on its perceived usefulness. That makes it also contingent on the perceiver.

Now, pretend you are a manager of a public mental health and addiction program. You have choices to make when the staff education requests start to come in. You need to decide, for each request, what its value or usefulness is. If your priority is that you want to satisfy the staff, then you will approve most or all requests, provided that the budget will allow it. This can easily be justified by saying that staff satisfaction is the priority.

If you were to take a client-centered approach, you would start with the assumption that the needs of the client outweigh the needs, or at least the desires, of the staff. You would recognize that staff engagement and satisfaction are important, but that your job is to help achieve it without doing so at the expense of clients. For every day that you send a staff person out of the clinical setting for a workshop or conference, you add another day to the collective wait time. You actually take publicly-paid, clinical appointments directly away from clients. You may work to rationalize that, but it can't truly be justified from a client-centered perspective unless the workshop has a high level of utility *for the client*. In other words, will clients benefit in any direct, observable, and important way by that staff person attending that workshop instead of using the time for appointments?

If you were to ask staff this question, it would not be hard to predict the answers. There are some common and predictable replies. They would talk about their thinking being stimulated, or about the general value to their clinical work simply from learning something different or new. Admittedly, all such intellectual stimulation is important and has value. However, it is not *as important as* directly serving the client (the public) that pays us. We may say it is a priority, but it is not **the** priority. It does not come prior to seeing clients who are in need of service. There are other ways to stimulate one's mind, many of which can be done outside of work hours. The taxpayer is not paying the program and its staff to engage in such curiosity-driven or personal-interest-driven cognitive stimulation.

If a workshop or training event is necessary in order to serve clients better, that is completely different. If it is a skill that is recognized as being fundamental to the delivery of the public service, then it makes sense to ensure staff have that skill. If it is learning about a new process, or a new way of doing something that is certain to directly and concretely improve the access and experience of the client, then it obviously must take place. In other words, we need to evaluate the level of utility of that education or training *to the client*. That is the issue that must be addressed.

People in management or leadership positions in a public mental health and addiction program must answer this on behalf of clients because they are the people whose interests the managers are paid to represent and protect. If any manager puts another person's interests before that of the clients, it essentially represents a failure to meet the primary obligation of the job. It is a violation of the public trust. Decisions need to be about the client first and foremost. *It's not about us.*

One way to address the issue of professional development is to ensure that all staff education and training is program-driven. At an individual level, if a person is identified as needing additional training in a specific area in order to effectively, efficiently, or compassionately treat clients, that training should be approved. Please note that this would be based on a collaborative decision between management and that clinician as part of a performance-management process. However, this should be rare. Presumably, staff are hired because they *already* have the skills to perform the job. Beyond that individual-targeted level, most of the focus on professional development should be to address gaps in the program's ability to meet clients' needs. For example, if implementing a new intake process, or a new model for improving clinical effectiveness, collective education should be provided for all involved in order to fill that gap. All such training has the purpose of directly improving the clients' experience or health.

There is also an important financial point here that specifically relates to the roles and responsibilities of a public service. Sending individuals to workshops and conferences is an expensive proposition. Having people come and do in-house training for the program's overall client-centered priorities is almost always more cost-effective. In a public service, there is an obligation to use tax dollars to serve the public interest. If a program is sending staff to conferences that are primarily just for general information-sharing and are, therefore, known *not* to change or improve the work the staff actually do, that is not in the public interest. If an individual staff member is approved to go to a workshop about a topic of personal interest for her own intellectual growth, but it is not a topic or skill *needed* for the job, then it is not an expenditure that is in the public interest. Technically speaking, in both cases the employee's needs or interests are given higher priority than the client in two ways. Tax dollars are spent that do not improve the program they are meant to fund, and clinical staff time is taken away from clients' access to service, thereby adding to the wait time.

In a public service, it is essential that the hard questions be asked. When people request to spend money and client time to attend an educational event, its *value to the client* must be considered, *without rationalization*. Will the education have a real, concrete, observable, positive impact on the experience or health of clients? Of course, many will say yes and be able to argue why their own intellectual stimulation makes them generally better at their clinical work. As I said, that is likely true. However, each of us in our jobs has a personal and professional obligation to keep ourselves on top of our game. It is not the taxpayers' responsibility to keep us learning things that don't help meet the mandate of the public program. Nor is it the taxpayers' job to keep staff intellectually stimulated. If the activity will directly improve an aspect of client care, by way of a clinician learning a new evidence-based clinical method, or a new process to help ensure smoother client access, then the value of that activity is higher and may justify the reduction in access that it causes by having staff attend.

Consider the value of staff education from the perspective of impact on the client. The more direct and significant the benefit to clients, the more value it has and the more appropriate it is to support it with tax dollars and client appointment time. Otherwise, it is putting things of less value before the primary needs of the client and the public interest.

Actions for system managers and leaders:

1. For all professional development activities, objectively assess the direct value to clients, without rationalization, and only spend from the clinical hours if there is direct and important benefit to the clients.

2. Plan professional development activities to be program-driven, specifically to improve the client experience and well-being, as opposed to spending clinical hours on curiosity-and-interest-driven education and training.

Actions for clients, supporters, and advocates:

Ask your local programs about staff educational events, benefits to clients, and amount of clinical time spent. Just respectfully asking will begin to create transparency on this public issue, and will therefore increase accountability for the funds and the clinical time to be spent in a client-centered way when it comes to staff education.

Barrier – Cancellations and No-Shows

For many years, both the mental health and addiction fields have been plagued with significant rates of cancellations and no-shows. A cancellation is when a client calls in advance of an appointment to tell the program that she is not going to be attending the appointment. A *no-show* is when a client does not contact the program with any notification, but then simply does not show up for her appointment. These appear to have been more frequently an issue in this program area than in other components of the health care system. There are a few key factors that likely account for most cases.

Let's begin with the simplest. Because wait times have been so long, people often forget their scheduled appointment. That day eventually comes and goes without the client even being aware because of the delay. A second likely cause is that, when wait times are long, a person's problems often escalate to such a degree that he ends up entering the acute care system (i.e., the emergency department and/or a hospital bed), making the original out-patient appointment both insufficient and redundant. The third key reason is that the longer the wait times, the more time people have to change their minds because of stigma, discomfort, anxiety, or perhaps even denial and rationalization. Finally, of course, there are many cancellations that are simply the result of conflicts in people's schedules and personal or work-related issues that come up, and that were unforeseeable many moons ago when the appointment was set.

It is reasonable to assume that if wait times were short and people could get in the same day, or within a couple days, or even within only a few weeks, the occurrence of these factors in people lives would decline. Therefore, the no-shows and cancellations to which these factors contribute would also be reduced. If someone calls and gets timely access when he decides he needs help, the shorter time frame reduces the probability of (1) his forgetting, (2) the problem getting worse and requiring acute care, (3) his changing his mind, or (4) scheduling-conflicts arising. We can hypothesize, therefore, that if we reduce our wait times to allow more-immediate access, we will have fewer cancellations and no-shows. That, in turn, will reduce wasted clinician time.

In the meantime, until we reduce or eliminate cancellations and no-shows, each one represents potential for another client appointment. We just need to get those hours into the bank of available time. We need to have processes in place that smoothly and efficiently reassign all these hours as they become available. The goal is to have no unused clinical hours. In this regard, cancellations are slightly different from no-shows because we have advance notice (even though it is sometimes only hours) that the person will not be showing up. For a no-show, we don't actually know until 10 or 15 minutes after the appointment time that the person is not arriving. The next two sections look at addressing each of these separately.

Cancellations

In order to maximize the use of all *cancelled* clinical appointments and ensure that clients benefit from that paid time, there first needs to be a centralized intake system by means of which intake staff control all the clinicians' calendars, as described earlier. The basic process after that is really quite simple. A procedure must be in place so that all cancellation calls go directly and immediately to the intake staff, not to the therapist. If they do go to the therapist, he needs to be required to forward the information *immediately* to the intake team. Timeliness, even minutes in some occurrences, is critical here. The intake team knows the clients who have been waiting the longest, or clients who have somewhat more urgent needs. When the intake team finds out about a cancellation, they are able to contact one of these clients, and book her into the cancelled slot.

If we have a high-functioning intake team, and a robust communication process, this filling of cancellation slots can be done even with very short notice. There are many clients who would gladly drop what they are doing to come for an appointment with only minutes or hours of notice. This can make an incredible difference in the amount of clinical time available, and can cause an observable reduction in wait times (cancellation and no-show rates together can amount to anywhere from 10%-30%, which amounts to a lot of available or wasted clinical time). In addition, immediately filling these slots does indicate that the program is working to make the clients' experience the best it can be by offering earlier appointments when they arise. That, by itself, will increase client satisfaction because the intention of the process is simply to do better for the client by not wasting any appointment time.

This will not necessarily be universally accepted by all staff. Most will understand and embrace this decision and will follow the procedure of reporting all cancellations immediately because it is the right thing to do for clients. Unfortunately, I have seen rare cases where an employee, who prefers to get the extra time for herself to work on other things, regularly fails to inform the intake team of a cancellation she receives, or *forgets* to tell them until it is too late to be rebooked. I know... that's appalling. But, if you look closely enough at the patterns, you will find these types of inefficiencies that are not the norm and not the practice of most staff, but do vary according to the person. There are very few people who could knowingly keep clients waiting in this way, but, once in a while, in one place or another, one or two such people do end up working in any program. That is why it is essential that clear reporting expectations be put in place in the standard procedure for dealing with cancellations, and some monitoring must be done.

If your mother were a client waiting to get into the service, how would you want this system to work? You would likely think that immediate and flexible rescheduling of a clinician's appointment slots should be the standard approach to prevent wasting that paid time from which your mother could have benefitted. This is simply about prioritization, and about running a system flexibly and responsively, rather than rigidly.

Actions for system managers and leaders:

Require, through policy and performance management, that the intake team always be informed instantly of all cancellations, and that they immediately (even if there is only short notice of hours or even minutes) attempt to fill that slot by calling and booking someone else who may have some urgency or may have been waiting a long time.

Actions for clients, supporters, and advocates:

1. If you have an appointment you need to cancel or reschedule, please call the program as soon as you can, so they can have time to schedule someone else into that time slot.

2. When looking for an appointment, and if wait times are long, ask your local program about being put on a cancellation list. If they don't have such a thing, advocate for them to start taking this approach to filling all cancelled appointment slots (even if at the last minute).

No-Shows

As previously noted, no-shows are clearly different from cancellations in that there is no advance notice. That does not mean the time can't be salvaged for clinical purposes. There is one primary way that this can happen. Often, it will be possible for the clinician to switch some time around during that week. For instance, there may be a time slot over the next couple of days where the clinician was scheduled to do some of her necessary administrative work, such as case notes, client phone calls, and client advocacy with other agencies. These are all important activities regularly scheduled into everyone's week. Now, let's recognize that a no-show time slot has no value to other clients *at that moment* because the appointment time has already started. Therefore, that time slot is only going to be good for administrative purposes. Future/planned administrative work could be done at that time. In other words, the administrative tasks planned for later in the week could be done during the unused clinical slot from the no-show. Then, the block of time later in the week that was scheduled for administrative work could be converted to a clinical appointment. The intake team could use its judgment, and fill that *new/replacement* clinical slot the way they would normally fill a cancellation (described above).

The key point is that instead of the clinician now having two administrative openings in the week in which clients will not be seen, she still maintains only one, but switches the day and time of it. The system thereby prevents a loss of capacity and an increase in wait time, simply by being uniquely and creatively responsive to each such unexpected no-show. If the clients are at the center of our system decisions, then we don't allow that client appointment time to get lost. We simply move it and switch it with administrative time.

As you may have already figured out, the challenge in this approach is that it requires complete flexibility and a high level of adaptability among all staff. It also requires clear policy and procedures to ensure the Intake team is informed of every no-show, switches the admin and clinical slots in the clinician's schedule, and then books a client into the new clinical slot. This may seem to the more rigid thinkers to be inconvenient and challenging, but everyone must be reminded of the most important point of all – that *it's not about us,* it's about the client.

Actions for system managers and leaders:

Establish a policy and procedure to ensure all no-show slots are switched with a future administrative time slot in the clinician's schedule, and then that new clinical appointment is filled immediately, so the client population being served does not lose that clinical time.

Actions for clients, supporters, and advocates:

Try hard to attend your appointments. Even if you can't, try to let the program know you won't be coming. Even if you can provide some very short notice, it helps other clients more than if the program receives no notice.

Barrier – Therapy Time Used for Long-Term Social Support

Earlier in the book, I mentioned that mental health and addiction staff often find themselves in very long-term, supportive relationships with some clients. Commonly, these are clients who have gone through therapy, achieved some goals, become much healthier, and now are not actively receiving what most would define as therapy. What they receive in their still-regularly-scheduled appointments is more like general social support and life coaching. That is great, and is a success story. However, it is using the wrong resource for the job, and preventing other people from having access to the program. If therapy is not currently needed, then why provide the services of a professional who is trained for therapy? Why not help the client build up a social support network with family, friends, support groups, and other community agencies? That is where the skills and long-term sustainable benefits of social support really exist. It is often and reasonably argued that we do harm to the client by creating and sustaining dependence on the therapist for such non-therapeutic support.

There are many people in our client population (the taxpaying public) who are in need of, and waiting for, an appointment with a clinical psychologist, social worker, therapist, or psychiatrist for appropriate psychotherapeutic or medical interventions. Any hours those professionals spend seeing clients for supports that are not psychotherapeutically or medically required are hours that could be made available to those waiting for service and becoming more ill. Such misuse of resources adds to wait times and reduces access.

So, what is the solution? Here are two suggestions that have had remarkable results and that, by themselves, dropped wait times by weeks almost immediately. The first one is to have staff pretend they are retiring or moving away. It is always fascinating to observe that, when this really does happen with a clinician and he wants to reduce how many clients he will need to transfer to someone else when he leaves, caseload reduction happens as a matter of course and necessity. With much greater ease than expected, with minimal therapist or client resistance or difficulty in most cases, clinicians are able to close 30% to 50% of their cases ethically, appropriately, and safely. Time slots for psychotherapeutic purposes/appointments can indeed be freed up if we focus on the purpose and function of a therapist, and use his time for that function.

Ask clinical staff to pretend they are leaving, and to close all cases that could appropriately be closed in that scenario. Ask them to assure clients that, if they have further problems, service will be made available, the same as they would if they were actually retiring. Then, give the clinicians a deadline to identify those clients and begin the discussions and case closures. Most will produce, without a problem, a significant number to close. A few will struggle with this task. Those few will require more direct assistance and involvement with a clinical leader/supervisor to complete the sorting task. But, it absolutely does work to immediately reduce wait times and increase access. It also ensures that those clients who are exiting services receive the right information, contacts, and supports that are needed for their own level of health, or they get redirected to another service or a more appropriate component of the same program.

Actions for system managers and leaders:

Request that clinical staff close cases that they would be able to safely and ethically close if they were leaving or retiring in a few weeks, and redirect those clients to a more appropriate level or type of service or program for their ongoing support. This will ensure that all clients end up better matched to the right level and type of service (and not over-served by seeing a therapist for general support).

Actions for clients, supporters, and advocates:

Don't accept the myth that once you are receiving therapy from a therapist it means this particular service is what you will always need. The goal of a good mental health and addiction program is to help you become healthy, independent, and require less-intensive services over time.

Caution – Valuing Staff Wellness

Many of these previous sections may appear to devalue staff members by suggesting strict management and use of their time. It is important to note that this is not the core subject of the book, and it has much written about it in other publications. However, there are a few brief points that need to be mentioned in the context of the client-centered approach presented.

The approach presented here values staff in a way that the current paradigm does not. It respects the fact that each has a specialty skill set, from paraprofessional counsellors to social workers, therapists, clinical psychologists, psychiatrists, admin support, managers, and health promoters. It prevents them from being undervalued or used inappropriately by having to deliver services for which they are either under- or over-trained.

This approach does not suggest staff should be prevented from looking after themselves (self-care for the care provider). It simply suggests that such self-care can be supported through vacation time, sick time benefits, flexible scheduling options, building a mutual-support team culture, employee-assistance programs, among others. It also suggests that, due to our obligation as a *public* service, it is simply not our right as a program to over-spend taxpayer dollars and worsen wait times in order to meet all personal needs of staff. All staff in all industries have a level of obligation to keep themselves healthy and able to do the job. For those challenging times, formal benefits like those listed above often exist.

This approach does not prohibit staff from doing the many required administrative tasks, such as collecting and recording data to satisfy the needs of the system. It merely says that such tasks, being less important than the client (if we claim to be client-centered), can and should be scheduled around the needs of the clients we serve, not vice-versa.

Workplace wellness is absolutely essential in this field. Clinicians often experience vicarious trauma, stress, depression, and burnout because of the emotional difficulty of the job. They need to be supported.

Managers and leaders need to build a culture that provides it. This can be done through open-door management for 'anytime' support, crisis intervention, mediation, opportunity to freely and safely vent and complain about changes, or even permission/direction to go home or call the employee assistance program for help. This can be done through common staff rooms where people can laugh, share, and even console each other. This can be done through the promotion of mentoring in the workplace. It can be done through managers always being open to input regarding directions and changes.

There are many established ways to help support the creation of a healthy workplace, and a healthy workforce. Those do not necessarily require that we place clients lower than staff in the prioritization process. It does not mean we have to increase wait times or waste our expert resources in order to achieve workplace well-being of staff. This is a job of finding the right balance, and historically, the paradigm our programs have operated within has been skewed away from the client being at the center. Through an effective leadership team (discussed in a later chapter), a client-centered paradigm as described here can be achieved while also maintaining a healthy workplace.

CHAPTER 9

GIVING CLIENTS A POSITIVE EXPERIENCE INSIDE THE SYSTEM

In the previous couple chapters, we discussed how to make the process of contacting the sometimes-elusive mental health and addiction system more client-centered, and how to help people get across the moat and into the castle in a timely and non-disruptive way. Making both those processes more client-centered will make a world of difference for those who have in the past felt like outsiders to a system that people have often found so hard to access. In this chapter, we look into what happens after someone gets in. We consider what the client does experience, or should experience, once she gets an appointment to receive some kind of care or intervention. What aspects of our systems and processes can we change to improve the client experience?

Serve Clients on Time

It is no secret and no overstatement to say that one of the greatest frustrations of clients in all of health care is showing up for an appointment on time, and not being seen on time. We arrive... and we wait. It might be five or 10 minutes, or it might be as long as several hours. It would be tempting at this point to jump off into a rant about how most services in the private sector would never survive if they operated like this and made their customers wait in this way. But, that is an often-used comparison that really gets us nowhere because it does not enhance our understanding of the problem within our public sector or our identification of practical, client-centered solutions.

Why do people hate this experience of waiting? Again, this is not complicated, but it is a question many clinicians or administrators do not think about often enough. So, once again, let's try to see things from the client's perspective. If it were your son or father who was the client, why would you dislike his having to wait for 10, 20, 40 minutes for a scheduled appointment? It is clearly frustrating, angering, and challenging to a person's patience. If we were to ask people more specifically *why* they consider such waiting to be wrong or inappropriate, what do you suppose they would say? What would you say if you were the mother of the client?

In such conversations, people often talk about feeling disrespected. They believe that their own time is just as important and just as valuable as that of the health care provider. They also often experience anxiety. They worry they will now be late for the next scheduled part of their day, or perhaps won't have enough time to pick up the groceries they planned to get in order to make dinner for the family. They worry about having to pay the daycare or the babysitter for an extra hour or two with money that they don't have. They feel anxious about getting back to work late, when they only have a certain amount of break-time or permission to be away from the job that day before having their pay reduced or their employment put at risk. This has very real and significant impacts on people's lives, and, yet, our system repeatedly fails to address it. We enter a contract with a client when we say we will see him at 2:00 on Wednesday, and then we violate that contract if he is not seen until 2:15 or 3:00. It is an organizational ethics issue.

This is reflective of the traditional medical model. The system evolved around the unquestioned knowledge and expertise of physicians, and people showed that reverence (and overwhelmingly still do) by bending and flexing and making their lives fit the schedule of the more important person in the relationship, the doctor. It was his time that was genuinely seen as the most important. The people who needed his help adapted. That is not a reflection on the individuals in the medical field, but, rather, it simply reflects the way the delivery of services, and the power difference between patients and physicians have manifested themselves in day-to-day interactions. It simply became normal. The systems and processes all center around the physician in the medical model, regardless of the empathy, compassion, and humanity of the actual doctors themselves.

Let's put this specifically in the context of mental health and addictions. The people coming for help are often there because they are experiencing problems such as anxiety, depression, or anger. Ironically, these are the very things that our programs then cause them to feel. Making them sit in a waiting room beyond their appointment time gives them more time to worry, or to experience increased social anxiety, or to feel anger. It gives them the opportunity and good reason to feel ignored, unimportant, valueless, and helpless, which are already part of many clients' traumatic histories or their current life-contexts. This is like an orthopedic clinic making potential knee-replacement clients wait on a moving treadmill. Our services are causing harm to clients in the very areas of their health for which they are seeking care.

It gets worse. We have known for decades in health psychology that waiting affects treatment (Meichenbaum & Turk, 1987). Specifically, the more dissatisfied a client is with her health care experience (e.g., because of factors like waiting a long time for an appointment date, or waiting to get into the office once she arrives on time for her appointment), the less likely she is to follow the advice of the health care provider. In cases of chronic illnesses such as depression and some anxiety disorders, this can greatly affect a person's long-term health. A client's willingness to practice new learned skills (e.g., stress-management), engage in self-management activities (e.g., exercise, refraining from alcohol, cannabis, and other drugs known to exacerbate symptoms), or even take her prescribed medication, is reduced. All this is at risk because our public service made her wait.

Clearly, all the people working in the system are not so cold and heartless that they would knowingly make people wait unnecessarily, or ignore evidence that this behaviour causes harm. Of course not.

Our problem is not an absence of good people, or a shortage of people with compassion who want to help clients. Rather, the systems in which these good people work *are not designed* to put the client first.

This last point gets us back to the earlier discussion about the way we use the word priority. Consider this issue of waiting from that perspective. If we have a client-centered service, meaning that the client is *the* priority above all else, then we would not let other things delay a client being seen. We can't claim to be client-centered and then let other things come before, or *prior to*, our commitment to the client. When discussing this with staff, it is not uncommon to hear responses like *"Yeah, but we have other important things to do too."*, or *"Yeah, but I also need to finish my clinical notes from the previous session."*, or *"Yeah, but sometimes I may be in a meeting that is running late."* Those *yeah buts* are again a major problem because they essentially constitute rationalization of non-client-centered processes and habits.

There is no disputing that those other job activities are important, just as staff so accurately identify. The question for the leadership of the program, however, is "How important are they when compared to keeping our promise to the client, and reducing the harm we would cause by making her wait?". Remember, priority is a relative term. We must choose what is *more* important. This requires setting a clear expectation that no other activity is more important than seeing a client on time if she arrives on time.

There is only one valid exception from a client-centered perspective. If a clinician is with a previous client who is in crisis, and termination of the session would be harmful, obviously there is an ethical obligation to address that client's urgent needs before seeing the person who just arrived. Other than that one situation, everything should be dropped when the client arrives. In a meeting? The clinician should leave it. Doing case notes? The clinician should stop and finish later. On a phone call? The clinician should tell the person they will need to continue the call later. Out for lunch and your food is not arriving in time? The clinician should leave and have her friends/colleagues get it as take-out for later. Compared to making a client suffer worse symptoms in the short-and long-term, as discussed above, none of these comes close in *relative* importance. They are inconveniences to the people paid to serve clients, who need to remember... *it's not about us*. It is about the client.

Actions for system managers and leaders:

Make and enforce policy that ensures a client will never wait if she arrives on time for a scheduled appointment, unless the clinician is dealing with a client crisis at that time. If that crisis is going to take a while, find someone else who is free to take the waiting client in for a conversation or a more comfortable place to wait.

Actions for clients, supporters, and advocates:

If you or a loved one have been made to wait after arriving on time, and it is harmful or uncomfortable for you, respectfully express your concern about that to the therapist or her manager, and request that it not happen in future.

Assess and Treat Only What the Client Identifies

As discussed, this field has a long history based on an 'expert' model, in which clinicians assess everything they deem appropriate at the beginning of the clinical relationship. Aside from the flaws in this expert approach related to the quality of the client-clinician relationship and the power imbalance, there has been a great deal of inefficiency caused, as well.

The traditional approach is for the client to be assessed for a wide range of issues, well beyond that for which he has requested help. It was always considered appropriate to conduct a comprehensive assessment to be sure the clinician knew everything that might be going on with the client. Let's imagine taking that same approach in another component of the health care system. You walk into an emergency department with what you believe to be a broken arm. The doctor orders a complete body MRI, blood work, colonoscopy, and so on. That would be absurd.

Clearly, this is a simpler example in which the broken arm will not have any significant inter-relationships with any of those things being tested. In mental health and addictions, there are often inter-related symptoms and experiences. Nonetheless, a client-centered approach would lead us to have a conversation with the client and allow him to determine what the focus of any assessment or treatment should be. This approach is more respectful of the client's right to self-determination, and also shows respect for the client's time. It shakes off the historical paternalism of the expert-driven, medical model. Finally, viewing the taxpaying public as our client, this approach is more appropriate because it does not waste clinician time on fishing expeditions (looking for things that are not indicated or asked about), when that time could be used to reduce wait times and give other people earlier access.

The older model is clearly based on the belief that the clinician needs to know as much diagnostic information as possible about the client. While that assumption is debatable when stated so broadly, the concept of needing to know certain pieces of information is not without merit. However, beginning the process with a focus on what the client explicitly identifies as the issue is the right thing to do, if we approach it from a client-centered value base. During the conversation, if another clinical issue becomes evident, there is no reason a clinician cannot raise that as part of the discussion and allow the client to have input into whether it needs to be assessed or discussed. If, of course, there is an issue of imminent risk, that must be addressed. But, short of that, our system needs to move toward respecting the client's self-knowledge and self-determination.

This shift resembles the shift that happened in the early days after Freud's approach of assessing and interpreting a client's unconscious dynamics. Freud proposed that the client had no way to access that information in the unconscious, therefore leaving the clinician as the only one who could find the truth. Carl Rogers held the view that the client knows more about herself than the clinician knows about her. That was a pretty dramatic contrast to Freud's approach. Our system's struggle to move beyond this expert-driven approach is quite problematic. It contributes to further disempowerment of the client, invalidation of her lived experience and of her self-awareness, and an erosion of her free will and right to self-determination.

In simple math terms, every hour spent searching for and assessing disorders and illnesses for which there is no indication, no client self-report, and no obvious symptoms, is an hour directly taken away from the access bank. It is another hour added to the cumulative wait time. So, under this traditional paradigm, a system can cause a client to feel disempowered and disrespected, while also adding to the wait time.

If the client were your daughter or sister, how would you want this to work? It is safe to assume you would not want her to have to waste hours answering what feels like a million irrelevant and odd questions. Perhaps, you would want her to be able to start talking right away about her own sense of her problems, concerns, or symptoms. Perhaps, you would want her to be only asked questions or given assessments for what she identified or at least what is clinically obvious in her symptoms. Perhaps, you would want her to feel heard, rather than simply assessed and judged. That would be a client-centered system.

Actions for system managers and leaders:

Establish processes and policies that ensure clients determine what gets talked about or assessed, and what does not. Unless there is evidence of imminent risk to self or others, respect the client's absolute ethical and legal right to have complete control and self-determination in this regard.

Actions for clients, supporters, and advocates:

Talk about what *you* want to talk about. The clinical session is yours, and the clinician has absolutely no exclusive authority to determine what will be discussed or assessed. Nothing can happen there without your consent. So, if you are not having a conversation about the things that matter to you, or if you are being asked a million questions in some lengthy standard assessment of everything, you can stop and change the conversation. It is your right.

Provide the Least-Intrusive Care Necessary
to Achieve the Client's Goals

The principle of least-intrusive care is one that has been around a long time across health care, and is spoken of regularly. It means just what it says. As a principle, it suggests that we should disrupt a person's life or functioning only as much as we **need** to in order to effectively treat his illness. Our level of intervention should always start with the easiest, least-painful, least-unsettling methods and only move on to harder, more-painful, more-intensive, or more-disruptive approaches if the earlier efforts are ineffective.

In our traditional paradigm in mental health, this is not always the norm. Many of the interventions that happen are actually the opposite. They are often far more intrusive, disruptive, or intensive than needed to get the job done. There are a few main phenomena that seem to cause this that we will discuss and for which we will consider examples.

The psychiatric paradigm, which is designed to look for and treat pathology and illness, contributes to many people receiving medicalized care who may not need it. A paradigm is essentially a way in which an entire issue is viewed and approached – a conceptual model and means of thinking about and responding to specific sets of phenomena. Western society has come to view this field as one that is primarily about psychiatric care. That comes somewhat naturally from media attention to extreme cases that involve hospitalization, resulting from the previously-discussed fact that virtually all the existing public-sector services are at the acute care end of the continuum. With the historical leadership in mental health never developing early intervention and less-intensive services for healthy people, this medicalized conceptualization has become normal. This is unfortunate because it leads logically to many people instinctively bringing their loved ones to a hospital for mental health care.

Going to a hospital makes sense in an urgent/emergent situation, especially where there may be risk of harm to self or others. Taking a person to a hospital is also appropriate if the need is medical in nature.

But, how do people know if their mental health or addiction issue is or is not medical? On what do they base that decision? Typically, they do not explore this question because all they want is to get help for their loved one. They want to go to whatever place they think will intervene and provide care. Since all they know is the societal norm of seeing mental illness as primarily medical in nature, and perceive or assume there is no accessible service of any other kind, they do what they know. They do what our psychiatric paradigm has created as a norm. They take their loved one to a hospital... to a medical facility.

In the context of least intrusiveness, this is out of step. Many people seeking help do not require medical intervention. Nonetheless, in the current paradigm, many end up being inconvenienced by waiting several hours at an emergency department, then undergo a significant level of assessment, when perhaps what they needed was to be able to get quick access to some individual or group counselling and therapy, or even peer support, to help with their symptoms. But, most of that doesn't exist in the public system, or is not accessible in a timely way. So, people use what does exist in this medicalized model, and experience more-intrusive methods than necessary to effectively provide the care they need.

For those who are experiencing more-significant and urgent risks, hospital care and psychiatric treatment is needed. However, we also know that many people who appropriately seek such care end up frustrated at the waiting times and at what is perceived to be a lack of responsiveness of the services themselves. Let's not forget the basic math we discussed earlier, which applies here as well. Given that our pathology-oriented system has never recognized the need to develop a robust and easily accessible early-intervention component, and many people end up by default seeking intensive and intrusive medical care through hospitals, it is no surprise that waiting will become an issue. For every one person seeking psychiatric care, who could be better served by a less-intrusive counselling, support, or psychotherapy service (if accessible), that is one more block of time taken away from a psychiatrist that could be used for those actually requiring psychiatric intervention.

This is nobody's fault. It is just the natural result of the way our medical paradigm has shaped availability of our programs. It is not because clients and family members are making bad decisions and going to the wrong place. They are going to the *only* place they know is open and available without booking ahead, perhaps for months. They are doing what any of us would do, and seeking care where it exists.

This is also not the psychiatrists' fault. They are merely seeing whoever comes their way through the emergency department or other access points. They do not control who the people are or what their level of severity or need will be. Nonetheless, the way the system currently functions is contributing to people being treated with more-intrusive methods than necessary because of the unavailability of the right services. This adds to wait times in emergency departments, adds to the inconvenience, stress, and disruption to clients, and is over-using the most-expensive care we have (psychiatric services in an emergency department).

This principle also has implications for inpatient services. Hospital units that provide mental health care, or withdrawal management services for addiction, often admit people for non-medical purposes, thereby providing a more-intrusive level of care than necessary. This is described in another chapter with regard to detox services, so does not bear repeating here in detail. Suffice to say that if a person's withdrawal process can be managed on an outpatient basis, her life should not be further disrupted by admitting her as an inpatient. That more-intrusive option should be reserved for those needing 24-hour, medically-supervised care because of dangers inherent in the withdrawal process – primarily in cases of severe alcohol dependence.

In mental health acute care units, a couple of related trends can be observed. One is that people have often been kept as patients for unnecessarily long periods of time (sometimes for years). This is partly due to having limited options of a less-intrusive nature available outside the hospital. A client may remain admitted because appropriate community-based supports are insufficient to continue his care after discharge. This flies counter to the principle of least-intrusiveness.

Additionally, people will sometimes end up admitted longer than needed (thereby experiencing more-intrusive care than required) because of public expectations. Consider this. As already described, the public accurately perceives the whole mental health system as being a psychiatrically-oriented set of services. They have not had enough exposure to the diversity and accessibility of all the other services needed across the continuum to tell them otherwise, or to meet their needs. Therefore, they have come to believe that hospital admission (even involuntary) is generally the *right* care. It takes on a sense of *one-size-fits-all*, or a sense that an inpatient service is the one that is somewhat universal and can/should apply to most or all clients. Because of the scarcity of non-medicalized early-intervention or less-intrusive services, this is often all the public knows. It is what our medical model has taught us. Therefore, when someone seeks help and is not admitted to an inpatient unit in a hospital, people are disappointed and even angry. The same often happens when someone is admitted but is then released after a brief period of assessment or care.

With a robust and accessible array of services that meet the diverse needs of the public (the client), we would begin to learn and trust that hospital-based care is not universally applicable. We would learn that there are more appropriate and effective services for the majority of people, and that the hospital units should be reserved for those needing that specific type of psychiatric care at the higher-level tiers. We would end up reducing the demand on the more-intensive acute services, thereby making them accessible to those for whom it is the right level of care. In a client-centered paradigm, the services fit the clients' needs, rather than all clients having to fit uniformly into the more-intensive medicalized kind of care.

Actions for system managers and leaders:

Build a robust and readily accessible support and early-intervention service that is convenient and non-medicalized, so people can receive the least-intrusive care appropriate for their needs.

> **Actions for clients, supporters, and advocates**:
>
> Advocate for better access to the less-intrusive, non-medical, non-psychiatric outpatient services that are more appropriate for most people seeking help for mental health and addiction concerns.

Ensure Smooth Client Flow and Collaborative Care

The word collaboration and the term collaborative care are exceptionally common at this time in our health care system. They are used to mean a variety of related things. Some refer to a kind of health service that has various types of professions co-located within it. In other words, it is used to describe a structure and arrangement of services. In other cases, it refers to a process in which various people or services share the care of a client. The following section addresses the latter of the two. It describes issues pertaining to the *way* clients' experience care when more than one health care provider, or more than one service, is involved. It reflects on this from *within* a mental health and addiction program, and, then, also considers the process *between* a mental health and addiction program and *other* components of the health care system in which it resides.

Collaborate within Mental Health and Addiction Programs

Across Canada, there has been a long history of public mental health programs and addiction services programs existing and functioning as separate entities, or at least separate and distinct government departments. As a result of this, formal processes and approaches evolved over time that had the ongoing effect of preventing collaborative care. Many of these have been based on long-standing beliefs and practices regarding confidentiality and anonymity.

Much of the formal addiction treatment field has its roots in the world of Alcoholics Anonymous, and many of the original staff had experienced recovery under that self-help model. The concept of anonymity became entrenched in the system, and was often used synonymously with the lesser concept of confidentiality. In any case, this most-restrictive approach to protection of client information inhibited communication with anyone about a client's needs. In mental health programs, there was an historical belief that we needed to strongly protect clients from anyone finding out about their mental illness. This was seen as crucial because of the perceived embarrassment, negative societal view of the mentally ill (stemming from the days of institutionalization), and risk of resulting social harms.

Both fields have evolved with this extreme belief about the need for privacy/anonymity. The extent of this belief and practice is not seen elsewhere in the health care system because, for the most part, other types of illnesses do not carry the same kind and severity of stigma (with the rare exception). The result is that these two closely-related fields grew up side by side, but oddly were like a brother and sister who for some reason were not permitted to talk with each other. This has seriously inhibited collaborative care and has prevented this area of the health system from providing client-centered service.

People experiencing mental health challenges often also have harmful substance use patterns, and people with addictions or high-risk substance use often experience some level of symptoms of mental illness. We could speculate all day about whether one causes the other, but all we would have is our speculation. Clearly, there is reason to believe that addictions can occur as a result of people self-medicating their anxiety or depression. Clearly, too, the harmful impacts and loss of control experienced by people with addictions can contribute to someone developing feelings of anxiety or depression. These kinds of inferences, based on our own anecdotal observations and reasoning, make some sense and are commonly-held beliefs.

From a methodological perspective, we must remember that much of our knowledge and many of our beliefs about this are based exclusively on anecdote and correlation. This means we can't conclude that one causes the other. Having said that, it is also important to consider that, from a client-centered service perspective, it doesn't really matter. Being able to say for sure that one of these experiences or illnesses causes the other is mostly an academic point. The part that affects our delivery of client-centered service is the knowledge that these two areas of illness often occur together. These days, this is referred to most often as concurrent disorders or co-occurring disorders.

The flaw in this terminology is that it is also focused entirely on the illness end of the continuum, or only at the top two or three levels of the tiered model. That fits perfectly within the traditional, pathology-oriented paradigm. However, it does not fit well within a client-centered paradigm because it completely excludes all those people who may be simply engaged in high-risk substance use, but who don't yet have a problem. It does not include or account for those who may be starting to feel sadness or anxiety, but are not yet ill. It does not include those who may have combinations of these early symptoms or behaviours because, technically, they only have concurrent *symptoms* and *behaviours*, not concurrent *disorders*. This is merely an extension of the arguments presented in the earlier discussion of prevention and early intervention.

Back to the main point. Our services need to be designed to provide the kind of support and treatment that meets each client's unique combination of needs. Our services need to eliminate the gap between the two historically-separate program areas. A client experiencing concurrent disorders or risk factors needs to be treated as a whole person, not as separate pieces. In a traditional model, someone would be seen by a mental health practitioner based on what was presented during intake. If it became apparent that the client was also actively, and possibly problematically, using psychoactive substances, a formal referral would be made to an addiction program. In addition, many such clients would be told that further clinical work on their mental health issues would have to be paused until they successfully stopped using the drugs. This was based on the assertion that we can't accurately assess a person's mental illness if she is using something that can affect her emotions and cognitions.

If someone came to addiction services presenting with an addiction-related problem, the therapist would use a combination of approaches.

Very often, she would provide therapeutic interventions for the substance use as well as the symptoms of mental illness, at least in the most common areas of depression and anxiety. However, if the client's condition was of a higher severity than the therapist was used to, a referral would be made to a mental health program to treat that part.

So, most often, when someone appeared in either of the separate programs, she would end up with double the appointments, double the health care providers, double the discomfort, and feeling as if she had two completely distinct and independent parts of herself being treated. Clearly, these kinds of issues are not so-unrelated as to justify that separateness of treatment. It is not like we are talking about asthma and a broken finger. Those are obviously distinct and require independent treatment, more so than harmful or risky substance use and experiences/symptoms of mental illness.

There is no question that the people working in our systems now fully understand the degree of relatedness of these issues, and the likely extent to which they are interdependent and reciprocally influence one another. The problem is that, under the current traditional model, our programs do not respond accordingly. The effective treatment of concurrent disorders/symptoms requires that a client engage with a singular system that comprehensively provides a single plan of care that is seamless, least intrusive, most convenient, most respectful of her as a whole person, and matches her unique combination of needs.

To achieve this, we must turn our attention to the way in which we manage the integration of mental health programs and addiction programs. If such integration is done well, with attention to the right components of inter-group relations (as opposed to just thinking of it as an administrative and structural process), then there is no need to put much focus on the issue of concurrent disorders. Client-centered and individually-customized work will naturally happen, along with all the consultation needed to make it simple and least intrusive for the client. The process of accomplishing this type of structure is described in detail in the later chapter on integration of mental health and addiction programs.

Collaboration with Other Components of the Health System

The high degree of structural and operational segregation and distinctness of public mental health programs and public addiction services programs has not only inhibited collaborative care between those two program areas (as described above). It has even more significantly prevented comprehensive and client-centered service by the health care system overall. Let's look at an example that has been problematic for decades, but in which we have more recently been making progress, primary health care. We will then also take a look at how this issue applies in chronic disease management and in seniors' care.

Primary Health Care

In the field of primary health care, family doctors have always regularly encountered clients with risk factors or symptoms of mental illness or addictions. Many physicians, to their credit, have taken the time and effort to learn the information and skills needed to effectively intervene and provide the support or treatment needed for those individuals. For those who have not, or for those cases severe enough to be beyond the physician's level of confidence, the local mental health and addiction programs have been relied upon. That, in itself, is not the problem. The problem lies in the way in which the systems have addressed that reliance and how they have operationalized the interaction between physicians and the mental health and addiction programs.

When it is determined by a physician that mental health or addiction issues need to be addressed by the public system, a referral form ordinarily would be filled out and sent to the mental health and addiction program. For decades, that has been the normal process, and, in fact, has been the only mechanism through which physicians have been able to share the care of a client with the mental health and addiction programs.

The program would receive the referral and, depending on local protocols, may or may not communicate back with the physician to confirm that they received the referral, or that an appointment had been booked. Another point of variability based on local discretion has been communication back to the physician about clinical findings, treatment approaches being used, or outcomes of the treatment. Very often, such information has not been provided back to referring physicians because of the extreme approach to confidentiality described earlier. The most common exception to this would be if a physician has made a referral specifically for a *psychiatric* consult. In this case, the psychiatrist, as per standard obligations of medical specialists, would communicate back the results of the consultation to the family doctor.

Under a more-current and comprehensive definition of collaboration, we would see these two kinds of health care providers working together (*co-laboring*) to provide care for the whole client. That is not what this previous process description illustrates. Instead, what it depicts is parallel work, or parallel treatment. In other words, the doctor is providing care for some aspects of the person's health, and mental health and addiction staff are providing care for another component of the person's health, but independently of one another. These two streams of health care go on without communication. They go on without the coordination needed to ensure *common* goals and approaches, or at least to prevent conflicting approaches. This may constitute simultaneous and co-occurring health care, but it certainly does not constitute collaborative care.

Over the past 10 or 15 years, there has been a very gradual promotion, acceptance, and adoption of a more-integrated, collaborative care model. This is evident in the fact that we have more and more primary health care clinics across the country in which mental health and addictions treatment staff are providing direct service. The type of collaborative model that is in place, and the nature of the interaction among the professionals providing each of these components of care, is quite diverse. In some cases, it is merely a co-location. That is, there is no unique or integrated kind of interaction. Referrals may still be happening in the traditional bureaucratic fashion, but the location where the therapist would see the client happens to be in the same clinic. In other cases, the model goes far beyond this parallel and segmented type of care. In those cases, it may involve a doctor or nurse practitioner and a therapist literally working together on the development and delivery of a comprehensive treatment plan.

Consider this from a client-centered perspective. If the client were your husband, how would you want this collaborative care to work? It would not make sense or feel very smooth to have it handled as a formal referral that is managed through separate processes of intake, wait times, booking, etc., when both health care providers are right there, supposedly working as part of the same clinic/team. You would likely want the doctor to speak with the therapist to get advice on how to manage your husband's care without his needing an appointment with a second health care provider. If his needs can be met by the doctor herself, with good advice and consultation from the therapist, why double your husband's number of appointments and amount of inconvenience?

Suppose your husband's needs were beyond what the physician could meet, even with consultation, and he did need to see a therapist for specialized support or treatment. You would probably want the doctor and the therapist to jointly identify what the best treatment plan is, rather than each one independently planning to treat part of him. You would likely want that process to be designed for his convenience. For instance, you may want him to be able to go to the desk on his way out and book one appointment time at which he could see the doctor and the therapist either together or back to back (if seeing both is part of the treatment plan). If you prefer your husband to be treated as a whole person, you may want the doctor and the therapist to be able to look into a single paper or electronic file and see what treatment each of them is providing (so they can always keep coordinating care and avoid treatments that are contradictory). In other words, you would want your husband to be provided with *collaborative* care, rather than *parallel* care.

That would be a client-centered approach. It would not be about convenience for the doctor or the mental health practitioner. It would not be about the desire or perceived need for independence of decision-making and care delivery by either profession. It would not be about the system's need to maintain independent administrative processes, like scheduling, client records/files, etc.

The health care providers involved need to remember *it's not about us*. It is instead about what is best, simplest, least intrusive, most comprehensive, and most convenient for the client. Simply put, a fully collaborative care approach between primary health care and mental health and addictions can and should be designed to be client-centered.

Additionally, it is also worth noting that there are many private-practice psychologists prepared to enter into this kind of fully collaborative partnership with primary health care. So, physicians who struggle to get quality collaborative relationships with a rigid public mental health program in their areas may still be able to move collaboration forward. They can talk with private practice psychologists in their areas about establishing or improving collaborative care. Even if the public system is not ready for such a relationship, collaborative care for clients in a primary care practice may still be possible.

Actions for system managers and leaders:

Integrate mental health and addictions staff into primary health care clinics to the fullest extent possible, so that they work as a team in jointly planning and delivering care for each client, and use single, integrated, administrative processes. This means giving up some ownership and control of the staff, the processes, and the independence of each health care provider's clinical decision-making.

Actions for clients, supporters, and advocates:

Encourage your mental health and addiction therapist, and your doctor, to talk with each other and work as team on your health care. They don't need to be located in the same building or the same program to work together and treat you as a whole person.

Chronic Disease Management

We have known for quite some time that there is a strong relationship between the experience of chronic disease and the experience of mental illness. Most of the evidence is correlational in nature. Our intuition and our observations would lead us to believe that being diagnosed with a chronic condition makes it more likely to experience depressive symptoms. The strong correlation means that this kind of causal relationship may in fact be possible. However, our intuition and observations also lead us to believe that experiencing mental illness makes it more likely for us to end up being diagnosed with a chronic condition because it affects our health-promoting or health-inhibiting lifestyle and behavioural decisions and habits. The correlational evidence again implies that this type of causal relationship is possible.

However, there is a third, equally likely, explanation for the correlational data. If someone's life is dominated by unhealthy behaviours more than healthy behaviours – regardless of whether it is because of individual choices, poverty, or environmental, religious, cultural, or corporate influences – the impact is the same. That person may be more likely to experience chronic disease and also to experience mental illness (especially anxiety or depression related to the direct or indirect effects of those behaviours on physical or mental well-being). The bottom line is that, even though there is a strong correlation, the nature of the research does not allow us to validly conclude that any one of these causal theories and observations is the main explanation for the relationship.

Having said all that, on a practical level, it really doesn't matter. What does matter is the simple fact that people with mental illness very often experience chronic diseases, and people with chronic diseases very often experience mental illness. It is, therefore, reasonable to focus our energy on collaboration between chronic disease clinics and mental health and addiction programs. They share many of the same clients.

If we look at this from a client-centered perspective, it would lead us to the same conclusion. If the client were your sister, would you want her to go to a cardiovascular clinic to help her with her heart problems, go to a separate diabetes clinic to help her with her glucose levels, and then also go to a distinct and separate mental health and addiction program to support her in managing the depression she developed in connection with those illnesses? Of course not.

Even if, in all health care jurisdictions in Canada, all chronic disease clinics were functioning in a fully-integrated way (i.e., a single, integrated clinic for diabetes, heart disease, asthma, COPD, etc.), we still would not want our sister to have to deal with the physical illness in one place and the psychological challenges in another, as if they were each completely independent. A client-centered approach leads us to treat the client as a whole person, and provide support or care for the full array of needs that each person presents or experiences. It leads us to think in an integrated way about services and to take down the walls. It leads us to stop thinking about these clinics and programs as separate entities that each need to manage their own clients, in their own way, in their own systems.

If we want to take collaborative care to the point of actually being client-centered, then psychiatrists in our mental health and addiction programs, being medical doctors, would be regularly involved in monitoring and supporting a person's *physical* health status while they are involved in mental health treatment. They would at least be monitoring (and potentially treating) the primary risk factors and symptoms of the most common chronic diseases. If we were to take collaborative care to the point of being truly client-centered, there would be mental health counselling and treatment expertise built into chronic disease clinics, through training of the usual clinic staff, and through mental health clinicians being located within those chronic disease clinics. But, remember, as noted in the previous section on primary health care, merely co-locating a mental health professional in a chronic disease clinic is not collaboration or collaborative care. It is just co-location. The quality, seamlessness, and integrated nature of the working relationship also matters, and they often are determined by the systems and processes put in place to support or inhibit those relationships. A client-centered approach would lead us to create quality collaboration between mental health and addiction programs and the chronic disease management programs and clinics that exist within the very same health system. That is what any of us would want our sister to experience.

Actions for system managers and leaders:

1. Work to have psychiatrists routinely monitor the symptoms and risk factors for the most common chronic diseases because their clients are more likely to develop such diseases than most people.

2. Locate clinicians within your local chronic disease clinics, and help facilitate a fully collaborative care relationship between these two staff groups, because those chronic disease clients are more likely to develop symptoms of mental illness (especially depression) than most people.

Actions for clients, supporters, and advocates:

1. If you are experiencing mental health problems, and seeing a psychiatrist, ask him to check and monitor some of the indicators of chronic disease.

2. If you are a client of a chronic disease clinic, ask them to work with mental health and addictions to establish a collaborative care relationship and treat you as a whole person.

Geriatrics, Seniors, and Continuing Care

As our population ages, we are starting to see more-frequent examples of seniors experiencing neurological and behavioural difficulties. This has created some tensions between types of medical professionals, and also between health care program areas. Depending on where you go, and with whom you talk, you will find some psychiatrists who believe they should not be involved in the care of dementia patients. They see that as the role of family physicians and geriatricians. They actively resist using mental health resources, such as mental health beds, for such clients.

On the other hand, staff in various seniors' care programs, family physicians, and families of the clients see things a different way. They require assistance. They want and need the expertise that psychiatrists have in terms of both neurology and behaviour. They sometimes need the safety of an inpatient unit that can be locked. They need the extensive and highly-effective skills of mental health nurses at managing, de-escalating, and redirecting people with cognitive and behavioural difficulties.

Unfortunately, the traditional silo of mental health services, under a psychiatric paradigm, has in many areas maintained the moat around the castle in this regard. These intentionally separate and independent components of our health care system often engage in a tug of war over who will and will not deliver care to such clients.

It is sad to watch this happen when a family is turning to what they think of as their single health care system to provide the right care. If our programs were separate entities, then you might expect such a tug of war. But, they are not. We have a single, publicly-funded, universal health care system. Everything else is merely semantics because it reflects nothing more than whatever organizational structures we create for our operational simplicity and convenience.

No program within the health care system in Canada should have the right to act as if it is an independent entity and draw such boundaries around their participation in the care of a client. It is a single, public health care system. It is a single client. We need the leadership to think as a single system, direct people to drain the moat around the mental health and addictions castle (and others in health care), and direct the system to use all of its diverse programs and resources *collaboratively* to address the needs of each client... and then serve the next one just as flexibly, uniquely, and compassionately. Each client will need his own unique combination of services and components of care, and each of our programs need to be prepared to do those things they have the skills and resources to provide. If the client were your mother or grandmother, how would you want this to work? We have one health care system, not several, so likely you would want her treated collaboratively by all the professionals and programs that have relevant and useful skills to help her.

Actions for system managers and leaders:

Involve mental health and addiction psychiatrists, clinicians, and nurses in collaborative care relationships with your local seniors' team, as well as continuing care programs and facilities. They have valuable skills to contribute to the well-being of these important clients who deserve our best collaborative care.

Respect, Accommodate, Value and Welcome Cultural Diversity

We have been taught that it is politically correct to promote and support social inclusion and to respect and accommodate cultural diversity by providing culturally safe and relevant services. If we are trying to create a client-centered system, this is more than political correctness. This is more than just a growing norm, or an ethical obligation. Instead, this is a practical issue. It is a reflection of, and a component of, client-centeredness.

Client-centeredness means we do what is uniquely suited to each client. It means customization. It means case-by-case service design. It means sometimes compromising on our systems' over-simplistic but natural administrative tendency to gravitate toward complete standardization. Finding the balance between those two (standardization versus case-by-case service design/delivery) is the tricky part, but our history would tell us that the individualized, case-by-case customization of services most often gets the short end of the stick when competing with standardization. It requires a greater flexibility of thinking in how policies and procedures are designed, so it is more difficult for administrators to understand and operationalize.

What is this thing called diversity that we need to respect and accommodate? It isn't a new or complicated concept. It is simply individual difference. It is merely the fact that individuals and groups of people have unique characteristics, backgrounds, perspectives, and needs that make them distinct from other individuals and groups of people. The way client-centered is defined in this book is completely compatible with that concept. In terms of definition and operationalization, what this book is proposing is that services need to be designed and delivered in a way that custom-fits the distinct and unique needs of each client (i.e., individuals and populations).

This may sound like an over-simplification. But, if we build a program that is genuinely and fully client-centered, we will *necessarily* have a system that is responsive to diversity. We will have made our decisions about administrative processes, hiring, translation services, staff training, etc., to accommodate great diversity. We will have developed such a strong sense of responsiveness, adaptability, empathy, awareness of our biases and stereotypes, and client-driven care among our staff, that everyone can feel as if they fit. We will have empowered our staff to know that they have the **authority** and **responsibility** to make exceptions to standards and policies in order to accommodate aspects of diversity not previously anticipated or encountered... because *it's not about us.* It is centered around the unique needs of each client.

Trauma-informed Care

It is well understood that a high proportion of people who experience addiction or mental health struggles have also previously experienced trauma. In recent years, we have seen a welcomed increase in our awareness of this, and increased attention to how this should guide our clinical work. In our historical paradigm, our system has not done well at this. That is merely because an expert-driven, medical model tends to create a power imbalance between patient and health care provider, and also a more directive approach to communication. This is not what is needed by, and may even be harmful to, people who have experienced trauma.

If we want a client-centered program, we must ensure that all staff understand the effects of trauma, and the most effective and appropriate ways to communicate and interact with those who have experienced it. This must include everyone in the program. This cannot only be clinicians. Clinicians need to be able to have a better understanding than others, as they may be dealing with the trauma-related issues directly in therapy. That is sometimes about their having the skills to provide therapy for trauma itself. That is a specific clinical competency that needs to be present if they will be directly treating people for trauma.

There is another, more-broadly-needed skill set. Many clients being treated for specific addiction or mental health concerns or illnesses come to therapy with their issues being contextualized by the trauma they have experienced. They may be in treatment for depressive symptoms, for instance, requiring evidence-based approaches like cognitive behavioural therapy, but the nature of the relationship with the clinician matters. The clinician must create a safe environment that appropriately fits the strengths and vulnerabilities of someone with a history of trauma, even when not treating the trauma itself.

The way such a client is communicated with by the intake worker on the phone, or the receptionist in the office also matters. Trauma-informed care requires that all our interactions with a client make him feel safe and comfortable, and avoid triggering uncomfortable emotional reactions. To do this, all staff must have an understanding of trauma. The concept of a client-centered system described in this book supports and is supported by a trauma-centered approach. Client-centeredness requires that everything we do is designed to fit the needs of the clients (individuals or populations). Being informed about, sensitive to, and supportive of clients' trauma-related needs is part of that. Given that we do not necessarily know which clients have traumatic histories, everyone in the program must have the knowledge, skills, and behaviours that make their interactions safe and comfortable for *all* clients in this regard.

Actions for system managers and leaders:

Train all staff to be aware of the effects of trauma, and to have the skills to greet, interact with, and treat all clients in a way that supports their potential trauma-related needs.

Prevent Conflict of Interest, So The Client Interest Comes First

A conflict of interest is a scenario in which a person experiences influence or pressure to behave in two different ways that compete with one another or are different from one another in their effect. In other words, it is when a person has reason to decide to do things in one particular way, but a very different reason to decide to do things in a contradictory way. In clinical therapy within a public service, this kind of situation has commonly existed and does pose a direct threat to the concept of client-centered service.

Consider this example. A public mental health and addiction program employs a number of therapists who, coincidentally, also carry out private practice outside of their publicly-paid work time. This is common. In addition, some of our public programs have a history of maintaining a list of private practices, so that if a client is looking for a private therapist for whatever reason, the public program would provide that list to help the client know who is out there. On that list will be some of the staff of the public program who also provide private therapy. Such a list would most often be wanted by a client who is looking for either more frequent therapeutic contact than the public service can provide, or alternative methods of service or treatment that the public service does not provide.

It is important to think about how these situations can cause conflicts of interest and how such conflicts of interest can put client-centered care at risk. A therapist who has a private practice that delivers alternate methods not provided by his work in the public system is constantly in a position to advise clients about what kinds of treatment are most appropriate for her needs. That means that he is in a position to recommend the same kinds of alternative treatment methods that he provides for profit in his private practice. This is, by definition, a conflict of interest.

This therapist has two separate interests each competing for control of his decisions and behaviors. His interest in the well-being of the client may cause him to recommend one type of treatment approach, but his need or desire for personal profit in his second job (private practice) creates a motive, or an interest, that implicitly pressures him to recommend a treatment method from which he can profit. This does not mean that he is lying or manipulating, or trying to do wrong. It simply means that his objectivity is compromised, and he does not have *only* the best interest of the client influencing his clinical advice.

It is a conflict of interest for any public-service employees to profit, directly or indirectly, as a result of their publicly-funded work. That means if, by any information-sharing or advice, the client of that publicly-funded therapist ends up also seeing that therapist in private practice, a conflict of interest has been at play and has influenced the course of that client's treatment. When a public-service mental health and addiction clinician also operates a private practice, the policies and administrative structures of the system must ensure that the existence of that practice, and the revenue potential, can never be permitted to cloud the objectivity of that public servant or affect client care. This is essential because if the profit motive of having a private practice were to influence the nature of a client's therapy, or the nature of the recommendations from the therapist, then the client's interests are not at the center. The therapist's interests are also playing a role in determining the course of treatment and ultimately the well-being of the client.

While this is sometimes a complex issue, good therapists with solid internalized understanding of ethical boundaries respect this issue and are cautious about this risk. It is, therefore, not difficult for the system to help eliminate or control this risk for the sake of keeping the client as the priority. To help address this, a public program should never provide lists of private practitioners, and should never provide recommendations or information about anyone in private practice. In most jurisdictions, this would be an unnecessary communication anyway because every regulated profession has its own website, on which it provides all the information necessary for someone to find a private-practice therapist. Therefore, staff in the public system need only direct people to the posted private-practice directories for clinical psychologists, clinical social workers, counselling therapists, and other relevant professions in each jurisdiction. Policy within a public mental health and addiction program must provide this direction to staff. The program policy also needs to be explicit in stating that no individual therapist will provide information to a client about any private practice. This includes prohibiting even an acknowledgement that he has a private practice because this can implicitly influence the client.

Finally, given that a public service has an ethical obligation to use only evidence-based clinical methods, program policy must prohibit all staff from recommending any clinical method that is not formally endorsed or recognized by the program as evidence-based. To recommend such a method can indirectly end up leading a client to that therapist's private practice. It also constitutes a violation of that therapist's responsibility while being paid by the public program. In that role, he is a spokesperson for the *public* mental health and addiction program, not an independent practitioner with total freedom to share his personal opinions about clinical methods. He speaks for the program and, therefore, can only endorse methods that are endorsed by the program. If we expect to truly keep the client as the priority, we must ensure that no therapist is in a position of having any personal, vested interest confounding his clinical objectivity about what is best for the client, or influencing advice that he provides *on behalf of* the public program.

Actions for system managers and leaders:

Set policy that prohibits staff from recommending any private practitioner, or any clinical methods that are not endorsed by the public program, as either can create a conflict of interest in how the client is advised, treated, and implicitly influenced. If there is a conflict of interest policy in your organization, ensure all staff read and understand it.

Actions for clients, supporters, and advocates:

If you are looking for a private-practice therapist, call or go to the websites for associations of Psychologists, Social Workers, or Counselling Therapists in your province. You should be able to find help there.

CHAPTER 10

Keeping Clients from 'Falling Through the Cracks' – Interagency Collaboration

Understanding Collaboration and Partnership

There is reportedly an African proverb that says "If you want to go fast, go alone. If you want to go far, go together." While this seems intuitive, most of us have had partnership experiences that have neither produced speed nor distance. Consider the following common scenario. Your community realizes, possibly because of some misfortune or recent tragedy, that our young people are "falling through the cracks". When people use that term, they are typically referring to the observation that, while some of our youth may be involved with multiple sectors and agencies (e.g., mental health and addiction, child and family services, justice, education), there are still gaps between these organizations that cause the young people's needs not to be met.

Many of those needs are of the type that do not fit neatly within any of the separate service structures. Take, for example, sexual health. Whose job is it? Given that there is evidence of effectiveness of education to prevent disease and unplanned pregnancy, it might be argued that it is the job of the school system. Because this is a health issue, it could be argued that it is the job of the health system. In addition, however, there are issues of law (age of consent) and issues of access to safe, stigma-free, and perhaps even anonymous support and prophylactic tools (e.g., condoms, birth control pills) that are often provided by community-based, non-profit organizations. So whose job is it? Arguably, it is not any *one* agency's job, but a collective responsibility.

The word *collective* doesn't simply mean that it is everyone's responsibility, so everyone should do it. It means it is a responsibility that we must jointly address in a collective way. Otherwise, we end up with one of two common scenarios.

First, the situation can evolve into all the organizations trying to do everything independently. In other words, the schools, the sexual health center, the formal health system all attempt to provide education, counselling, access to medical services, access to condoms, and other related supports. No rocket science is required to understand this is inefficient and not collaborative.

The second, and perhaps most common, scenario is that each of the organizations puts a clear fence around its own turf, partly to keep others from doing their work, but mostly to keep themselves from going outside of their own mandate. In such a scenario, organizations spend a great deal of time and conversation focused on defining the limits of their respective mandates. Many public-sector services work hard to make sure the lines between the various agencies are thick black lines. In other words, much of the focus of each organization or department is on what they *can't or won't* do. This same approach is also common among departments within the formal health care system.

Besides some flexibility of mandate for the collective good, discussed a bit more in a later section, there is also a need for us to examine our own agendas and self-interest. Consider the following scenario. Pretend you are leading or managing a mental health and addiction program. You get an email one day inviting you to an interagency meeting with your local child and family service agency. You immediately see this as an opportunity because you know you could work better together if only they were aware of how *their* policies and procedures could be improved to be more compatible with yours. This is going to be a very useful partnership. Little do you know that they called the meeting because they were thinking the same thing about you and your program.

When the meeting takes place a couple things end up clear, at least to those who are open-minded enough to examine the dynamics objectively. First, neither agency came prepared to change its own practices and policies. This is evident when suggested improvements are raised or creative ideas shared, and the response is very familiar and very frustrating. The most common phrases by both organizations at the end of each great discussion about what is needed are along the lines of "There's no way we'd be able to do that.", "That's not the way our process works.", or perhaps "We don't have any more money." The second thing that becomes obvious is that there will be no significant changes made today for the clients.

The following sections describe a principle-based, client-centered approach that our mental health and addiction system can use to create effective partnerships that actually lead to change for the people we serve. When these key approaches are followed, amazing things happen for the clients and communities.

I Am Here to Fix Me, Not You

Let's take a look at what has happened in the scenario described above. First, each group came in with the perspective that this was an opportunity to improve what the *other* agency does. People may not even realize they are doing this. However, if you watch and listen to the conversations in any such interagency or interdepartmental meetings, you will hear many people either tactfully or abruptly asking questions about possible changes or improvements to one of the *other* agencies. When everyone comes in with that perspective, there is nobody present with the intention or preparedness to consider imperfections in their own work that require change. This missing piece is sometimes referred to as being self-critically-reflective. It is a process through which we honestly examine our own work and that of our agency with the intention of finding imperfections and areas to improve.

For interagency or interdepartmental partnerships to work, all the parties must be prepared to embrace the concept of self-critical reflection from the beginning to the end of the partnership. So, what does this mean in practice? It means that when we walk into a room with members of another department in the health system, or with representatives of other agencies in our community, our primary focus must be on improving our own program or agency. It means we do not look to change what someone else does. We focus on what we control. We focus on what we can change that will improve the experience of the clients we all serve. We encourage and welcome feedback, comments, and suggestions from others that can help us become or remain aware of what we can do better.

In order to achieve this, we need to leave our egos at the door. True collaboration in a partnership cannot happen and cannot thrive without a great deal of humility among the collaborators. When we establish our partnerships, we must start with the basic fact that each of us can only change or improve the things that we each respectively control. We do not actually control, or even fully understand, the other's world. However, we do each know the politics, processes, funding, staffing issues, public demand, etc., related to the programs or services we manage or represent. We can each, therefore, make decisions and changes to improve those areas that are our own.

At the same time, every other person around an interagency or interdepartmental table knows all of those same contextual pieces for *their* own area, and has the ability to make improvements. The implication here is that we need to shake off the traditional approach to partnership, which often is about looking to the other as the solution to some of our own problems, or working to keep from adopting more work from those other organizations or departments (e.g., "That's not our job.").

Intuitively, this sounds simple and rational. However, very few people are even aware or likely to admit that they enter such partnerships with the focus on changing others' practices and on defending their own. This is a common social psychology phenomenon known as a self-serving bias in our attribution processes. Essentially, we attribute failures or difficulties in our services to external factors, while attributing successes or positive behaviours or attributes to internal factors. This helps us maintain a positive sense of esteem at an individual (or, in this case, organizational) level. Such self-serving biases inhibit humility because they deter us from focusing critically on our own work, and our own achievements and failures.

When we develop our partnerships, we must build them very heavily around humility and self-critical reflection. We must specifically structure the relationship around a focus on finding *our own* flaws, imperfections, and opportunities for change and improvement. To paraphrase part of a speech by John F. Kennedy, *ask not what other agencies can do for yours; ask what your agency can do for others*. Remember, your goal is to improve the client experience, and so that means humbly, intentionally, and constantly, looking for ways to improve what **you** do, even if it means going outside your mandate or changing something about your service that you thought was good. *It's not about us.*

This perspective is incredibly powerful in a partnership. Its power is derived from three specific phenomena. First, and most importantly, it feeds us information (from the other agencies or departments) about how we can improve what we do, which gives us opportunities to constantly make our own services better for the client. Second, it creates reciprocity among the agencies. If you set the culture of a partnership around your offer to change and improve your own services to be more supportive of, and collaborative with, other services and agencies, they will do the same. It precludes a tug of war because everyone is offering not asking. Everyone is giving, not taking. Everyone is demonstrating leadership, not criticizing other leaders. In such approaches, a norm of reciprocity takes over. Third, it builds a relationship of complete honesty and absolute trust among the partners because there are no hidden agendas, there is no turf protection, there are no defensive reactions, and there is no posturing. There is merely an attempt to throw all the wisdom and resources together on the table to collectively help the people we are tasked to serve. It creates a collective sense that *it's not about us.*

Besides personal and organizational humility as a prerequisite for this approach, it is also essential that we have a high level of self-awareness and emotional control. These, of course, are aspects of emotional intelligence and there is much written about that construct. In the current context, there are two specific aspects of it that are essential.

First, we must be sensitive to and aware of the sometimes naturally-occurring negative or defensive emotional reactions we feel when our own work or the work of our program is implicitly or explicitly criticized. We need to be self-aware enough to know when we are feeling those reactions. Second, we must have the ability to override those emotional reactions and replace them with the rational exploration of the criticisms or suggestions we receive, simply for the sake of improvement. In other words, we need to control those emotions, and see this as an opportunity to genuinely explore ways to use those criticisms to improve the well-being of our clients. Without both of these skills among the partners, dysfunctional reactions will arise and compromise the trust and openness on which the partnership is built.

If the client is truly at the center, is the top priority for all agencies, and if *it's not about us*, then it becomes easy to collaborate in this way.

Actions for system managers and leaders:

Go into interdepartmental or interagency meetings with the sole objective of genuinely finding ways to improve *your own* program and services, not everyone else's.

Decision-Makers Only

The second major issue here is that people need to be willing and able to make decisions, right there at the meeting, to support collaborative progress. This requires that they have a level of authority to be able to make changes and revisions to the services or programs they represent. For this reason, front-line staff are not the best choice to send to interagency partnership meetings, unless the purpose is clinical.

In a previous chapter, it was noted that clinical staff attendance contributes to wait times, but that is not the reason being highlighted here. Front-line staff rarely, if ever, have the system, policy, financial, or political knowledge, or the delegated authority to be able to make decisions to proceed with program changes. If the discussions are going to involve or require self-critical reflection about what can be changed in the mental health and addiction program (as opposed to someone else's organization), then someone in management who has the authority to commit to changes must be present. Otherwise, great discussions take place, and then people go away from the meeting with nothing more than promises to consult with management and report back at the next meeting. Rarely does this lead to changes because of time delay, loss of momentum from the conversation, and the fact that the manager who then is consulted by the staff person does not have the full benefit of the interagency conversation that led to the proposed change.

Actions for system managers and leaders:

Unless it is a clinical meeting, ensure that the only people attending interdepartmental or interagency meetings are those who have broad system-knowledge and the authority to make improvement-oriented decisions and changes right there at the meeting without needing to wait for the approval of someone higher up.

Empowered Management

Obviously, even for a management representative attending interagency meetings, there are some kinds of changes that are of such a broad and significant scope that higher-level approval is necessary and appropriate. However, there is a great deal of day-to-day operational procedure that many lower and middle-management people should be perfectly capable of addressing through change-oriented decisions on the spot, at the meeting. For anyone working in management in an organization for which that is not the case, that is unfortunate.

For anyone who is in a management or leadership role in an organization, but yet is not explicitly empowered to make decisions and changes that improve services for the client, in the context of such partnerships, there are bigger problems than this partnership. It likely indicates that they are in an organization that lacks competent and secure leaders, and, therefore, they may not be the appropriate representative to sit at the partnership table. Being there, but being explicitly required or implicitly expected to check decisions with the boss first, is of no real value to the partnership. It leads to the same old time-wasting processes that never leads to change for the client or genuine collaboration among agencies. This concept of empowering members of the leadership team in a mental health and addiction program is discussed in more detail in a later chapter.

Actions for system managers and leaders:

Explicitly empower your managers and leaders to be able to make decisions and agree to changes while at interagency or interdepartmental meetings, without checking with you first. They have been put in a management or leadership role, so now trust them, and allow them to do what is best for the client, whether or not it is what you would have done if you were at the meeting.

Actions for clients, supporters, and advocates:

If you know of members of a mental health and addiction management team who do not have the ability to make improvement-oriented decisions and changes while at interagency partnership meetings, help advocate with more senior people in their organization for them to be given that ability. It will make a huge difference in the development of collective, client-centered care of the people the agencies or departments share.

Actions and Decisions Only

Another common limitation of interdepartmental or interagency partnerships, in terms of improving the experience of clients, is the extent to which meetings are based on *talking* versus *doing*. Many such meetings involve a great deal of information-sharing. Organizations and programs meet with the purpose of becoming more collaborative and working better together. But does that really happen? Let's look at a common scenario.

You arrive at the first interagency meeting. The organizer of the meeting begins to talk about the reason for pulling people together, emphasizing how much better we could all do in serving the public if we worked collaboratively. After some exciting conversation about the possibilities, the conversation soon turns to a discussion about developing *terms of reference*. This is a document that spells out who the members are, how often the meetings will be, who will chair the meetings, what the principles and values of the group will be, and what the overall purpose and desired outcomes will be.. It is really just what the group stands for and what the rules are that the group will follow. When the creation of terms of reference is mentioned, the experienced people in the room are suddenly flooded with a feeling of dread. This is not because they don't believe in constructing terms of reference for such a group. It is because they have been down this path before and realize that the construction process for such a document may be enough to kill the initiative by itself. They are about to enter 'wordsmithing hell'.

For the next several months, a portion of every meeting ends up dedicated to reviewing the latest draft of the terms of reference. At each such meeting, because there will be some variation in who was able to attend, components of the document you thought were agreed upon suddenly are revisited because someone is present who missed that last meeting. As the meetings unfold month after month, and the terms of reference continue to be a topic on the agenda for fine-tuning, the group begins to do other business despite not having finished the document that determines what the business of the group actually is. In such situations, we tend to gravitate toward what we know.

In this case, there are three things we typically know. One is that we each have information about our own programs and services, and we see this kind of situation as an opportunity to share such information with other agencies or departments who *should* know about it. The second is that we have an interest in knowing what other agencies are doing so we are, at least initially, happy to listen and learn. Finally, we each know what our preconceived ideas and beliefs are regarding what is wrong with many of the other programs and services. As noted earlier, we come in with our own sense of what some of the other agencies need to do in order to improve service to our communities and linkages between our agencies. We can end up, therefore, in conversations that either directly or indirectly point out those flaws. When this begins, the tension builds in the room and the sense of collegiality dissipates. By the time the first few months have unfolded, and perhaps the terms of reference are completed and approved, a number of the members have begun to have attendance problems. No surprise.

For some, this has become an issue of being bored and unproductive. Once the members have heard the overview and an update or two from the other agencies, there is very little else to learn (unless the meetings were six or twelve months apart). For these people, regular information-sharing feels futile. Therefore, it becomes hard to find a justifiable reason, in the context of a very busy schedule, to attend these meetings instead of getting real work done. When people have busy jobs in management and leadership, they must constantly decide which things they can afford to put time into because they can't do it all. It ends up, therefore, being a choice of which meetings and activities produce the best results or get the most accomplished. A meeting of repetitive information-sharing, built into the standing agenda as a *round-table*, or *check-in*, or *updates*, will quickly move to the bottom of the priority list for many people in leadership roles.

For some, this is more than just an issue of being unproductive. In every geographic catchment area, some agencies or programs are more commonly the target of criticism and suggested improvements by the public and by other organizations. If you happen to manage one of those programs, interagency meetings become stressful. Your relationships with people in the room are always riddled with tension. In conversation after conversation, you live with the expectation that something will eventually be blamed on your program. Someone will think they have the magic answer to fix the system that you happen to represent. Perhaps even worse, when such conversations come up, people sit in silence when you know they are having those kinds of thoughts. In any case, does that sound like a meeting you want to keep attending? Not likely.

So, let's assume we have reached the end of the seemingly-perpetual construction of terms of reference. What has really happened so far? Too much time has been spent trying to get this document perfected and agreed upon. In other words, too much time was spent discussing and documenting what we will do, and how and when, instead of actually doing any real partnership work for the clients or communities we share. In addition, at every meeting, a great deal of time was spent with agencies or departments telling each other what their own programs are doing, independently. Talk, talk, talk.

What do we all want from interdepartmental or interagency partnerships? Why do we keep engaging in them? Why do the clients and the public want us to work in partnerships and coordinate our work better? Why do so many organizations' strategic plans and mission, vision, and values documents contain reference to partnerships? Obviously, we tend to believe they have value. However, from a practical perspective, it can be argued that partnerships have very little if any *intrinsic* value. In reality, they have value *only* to the extent that they can produce results that would otherwise not be possible, or that would otherwise be more difficult or less efficient. In the example described above, these points are not clear. We get caught up in the myth that a partnership is an end rather than a means. It is not. It is *not* an outcome or a product. It is a *tool*. It is a collective way of achieving outcomes, or achieving system changes that will improve outcomes for the clients and communities we serve. Therefore, if all that is happening is talk, and things within and between programs are not actually changing or improving, then this is not a partnership that has value. It is just an information-sharing discussion group, and an enormous waste of human and financial resources... mostly taxpayers' money.

Partnerships should be intentionally structured around the simple rule that all agenda items and all conversations must be designed to lead to, and result in, a decision or action. Any item suggested for the agenda should be justified as action-oriented. Every conversation that happens at the meeting should be time-limited and enforced by the chairperson. Such conversations should be concluded with "So, what is the decision or action from this item?" If there is no answer to that question, then it was merely an information-sharing item and probably should have been excluded from the agenda and just emailed to everyone as a FYI (i.e., For Your Information). No discussion should ever conclude without an action or decision that moves something forward within the partnership that will benefit clients. When this approach is taken, the members actually attend meetings with incredible reliability and passion. They engage in more directed and purposeful discussion. They complete the actions they committed to at the previous meeting. They do not get bored. This becomes one of the meetings they actually look forward to attending.

It is possible to make such partnerships effective, but it requires intensive and intentional facilitation that constantly attends to all the issues described in this chapter. A standard approach by a chairperson in such situations **will not suffice**. This requires focused and skilled facilitation by someone who identifies strongly with such action-oriented principles and approaches. It requires constant assertive diplomacy to keep all emotions and defensiveness in check. This focus cannot be allowed to wane, even for one meeting because, when it does, the group often gravitates immediately back to information-sharing, critiques of one another instead of themselves, and feelings of being either unproductive or attacked. The selection of a chairperson, therefore, must be based on that person's strong facilitation skills.

This approach is unquestionably productive because things do actually change and improve, both within and between the organizations.

Actions for system managers and leaders:

1. Restrict all interagency meeting agendas to include only items that are action-or decision-oriented, with no allowance for items that are merely information-sharing.

2. Select a chairperson based on proven skill at facilitating and controlling the flow, action-orientation, and productivity of meetings, not just on democracy or rotation among members.

Small and Focused

Many people who have been part of a multi-agency or multi-departmental committee have found themselves sitting through lengthy discussions that were only relevant to a specific two or three of the many member-organizations present. This is yet another common reason for people and organizations to become disengaged from so-called partnerships, and for the cracks between agencies to remain unchanged. When that happens, as with the other causes of disengagement described in the previous sections, clients and communities suffer. They experience inconvenience, slower access, more-formal bureaucracy, less-smooth transitions, and very little true collaborative care. The systems don't actually become collectively client-centered.

We need to build partnerships that are small, limited in membership, and with a very focussed scope and purpose. It is recognized that this may sometimes mean knowingly excluding other agencies that may have been able to benefit from, or provide benefit to, such an initiative. However, the intention of this kind of partnership is to put a concerted effort into addressing the very important and reciprocally-influential relationship between two key partners to ensure real progress for their shared clients. That singular, common focus between only the two agencies guarantees that there could never be a conversation that is irrelevant to anyone at the table. With only two partner organizations present, there are no other relationships that can be discussed at such a meeting. It guarantees significant engagement and passion for the collaborative work.

It ensures, because of fewer people present, the building of deeply meaningful and trusting relationships among the participants. The value of that cannot be overstated. Because of the significantly sharper focus, greater relevance to the members, and higher action-orientation, it also justifies and benefits greatly from having multiple leaders from each organization attending the meetings. With that kind of larger representation, the ability to make significant decisions right on the spot increases dramatically.

It is important to note that, by taking this approach, programs and agencies may end up with more partnership meetings to attend. This can be inconvenient and time-consuming. However, when the productivity of the partnerships increases and causes real system change and real collaboration, as opposed to information-sharing and parallel work, it is well worth the time and effort. In other words, when it genuinely makes things better for clients and communities by virtue of being a more effective model of change-oriented partnership, that is what matters most. If we are client-centered, then our own inconvenience in attending more meetings is a lower priority than creating better collaborative services for the clients. *It's not about us.*

Actions for system managers and leaders:

Create small, precisely-focused, inter-agency or inter-departmental partnerships, between only two or three significantly-relevant, partner organizations rather than, or at least in addition to, larger multi-agency groups. Use them intentionally to build deep, trusting, change-oriented, client-centered, collaborative relationships that are less easily, less certainly, and less often achieved in the larger group context.

Frankness – It's Not About Us, So It's Not Personal

In many of our social agencies, and certainly in health care, honest and direct communication is rarely appreciated. More often than not, it is taken personally and perceived as aggressive. This frequently leads to the social psychology phenomenon of *groupthink* (going along to get along – putting group cohesiveness above productivity and honesty). People become bobble-heads who mostly just agree with others in order to avoid the tension that can come from disagreement. In our partnerships, we need to make sure that this type of culture is not allowed to develop. We must be explicit in our understanding, and in our terms of reference (when we break the norm and complete them in one or two meetings at most) that we will be direct and honest in our discussions, and that we will accept that directness and honesty from the others at the table.

The true secrets to understanding and being able to create this type of productive culture are in understanding and remaining steadfastly focused on the purpose for the partnership (the clients), and remaining focused on how to improve our own programs, not those of others (noted above). When we keep this client-centered focus, and this self-improvement focus, interesting things happen. First, no comments are ever intended to be, or perceived to be, aggressive, personal, or adversarial. This is because it is well understood and agreed that every statement or question has client well-being as its rationale and as its goal. This is also because we each intentionally choose to welcome all negative or critical comments as opportunities to improve our own work for those clients.

Another phenomenon that occurs as a result of this approach is that members of the partnership begin to feel safe engaging in the toughest of conversations. They don't hesitate to say what they are seeing or experiencing, regardless of its nature, for the sake of the client. Key issues that have been underlying the interagency relationships for years, but never addressed (other than perhaps in the odd passive-aggressive or back-room conversations), suddenly become appropriate, comfortable, and extremely productive conversations. Everything becomes an exciting opportunity for improvement, not an unwelcome suggestion or disagreement. From a truly client-centered perspective, there is no need to tip-toe around such issues. There is only a shared need to recognize the discussions are not personal, and are solely and objectively intended to identify and do whatever it will take to improve the well-being of the people we serve, because *it's not about us*.

Actions for system managers and leaders:

Create a culture in your interagency meetings that does not tolerate groupthink. It needs to be a culture that instead **insists on** honest disagreement for the sake of objectively identifying what is truly best for clients, and **insists on** members never taking such disagreement personally.

Allow/Encourage Overlap Between Mandates

Falling through the cracks. As noted, that's the phrase that is used often to describe gaps in public services. It is usually referring to the fact that there are components of service missing at the points of intersection between agencies or between departments within an organization. This results from organizations and departments being too acutely aware of, and sensitive to, the line where their mandate ends and the line where another's mandate starts. It is important that we begin desensitizing ourselves to that line. It is an avoidance of straying outside of our formal mandate that keeps allowing gaps to exist.

The solution to this problem is that we expand what we believe collaboration is, and intentionally allow each program or organization to stray outside of its main job and create overlap with one another's work. In such an approach, there cannot be a gap. However, this requires a flexibility of thinking, and a comfort with a grey area where we are used to having black and white lines. If we want to make our collaborative partnerships to be centered around the client, then we must be able to tolerate the amount of grey needed to ensure no gaps exist between programs. A client can't fall through a crack if there is no crack.

Unfortunately, there still exists some of the rigid, old-school thinking that creates the gaps. For example, I recently had a conversation with a leader in a public mental health and addiction system about suicide assessment and screening tools. This part of the conversation was about the help that non-mental-health-staff in the health system needed in identifying suicide risk. These staff would include, for instance, nurses in the emergency department or nurses on a medical floor. These are staff who sometimes come across individuals presenting suspected suicide risk. The staff need some way to help identify which cases require a psychiatry consult or involvement of a mental health crisis team. It had been suggested at this meeting that our program staff (the experts) would be the appropriate people to identify the best screening tool, and train the staff in those other health care departments on how to use it.

In the discussion about this issue, it was fascinating to note that one of the leaders in the mental health system responded to this idea by saying "That's not our job. That's *their* responsibility." – referring to the medical units and the emergency departments. It was not recognized that, in a single health care organization, building capacity for suicide screening across the whole system is the responsibility of the program that has such expertise – namely, mental health and addictions. This is a classic example of a situation in which people fall through the cracks because of an inconsistent or limited understanding of the concepts of collaboration and collective responsibility. Black and white lines that define turf serve to keep the system from functioning as a whole. Interestingly, if the mental health program wanted to buy automatic defibrillators for use in its own offices (in case of emergency), that same mental health leader would probably expect someone from the emergency department to help select the best machine and teach our staff how to use it.

If we come at this from a client perspective, the answer is really quite simple. When we go to a hospital, we want and expect the professionals and departments of that organization to be each contributing appropriately to our care, as a team. We expect that, if we have multiple kinds of health problems, the nurse, cardiologist, radiologist, psychiatrists, psychologists are all supporting one another's work by contributing their own expertise to collectively treating us. However, for this to happen in a client-centered way, the various components of a system need to know what their job is, but then be willing and committed to being flexible at the points where their mandate intersects with that of another service.

This same concept applies between public-service agencies and community organizations. Flexibility at the edges of our mandates is a two-way process. It doesn't just mean that we need to play nice or be careful at the points where we intersect with other agencies. It literally means that we need to be willing to go outside our formal mandate and allow other agencies to come inside our formal scope of responsibility if that is what is necessary to provide a genuine, client-centered experience for the people we jointly serve. If the mandates are allowed to overlap a bit, that is the way to avoid the existence of *cracks* that people can fall through.

We must move past this individualistic or silo-focused thinking. We must recognize that we do not have separate mandates among our health care departments, our community agencies, and our other government programs and organizations. As part of the taxpayer-funded public sector, we have one collective mandate. Our job is to look after the safety and well-being of our population, using whatever combined skills and resources we have. Regardless of what public-sector program or organization any of us may work for or support, we must remember… *it's not about us.*

Actions for system managers and leaders:

In our partnerships with other public-sector organizations or other departments, start promoting and internalizing the idea that we are a collective with a shared mandate from the taxpayer to look after the well-being of the public. Ignore the separateness of sub-components of this overall mandate, as much as possible, to allow for overlap and genuinely collaborative work filling the gaps between us.

Actions for clients, supporters, and advocates:

If you ever experience a mental health and addiction program indicating that a particular service or support, which seems to fit its mandate, is not part of its job, ask whose job it is. If the answer is unclear, you have discovered a gap. Advocate with your local program and with other local organizations to work *collaboratively* to cover that gap by stopping the old-style rigidness about who does what.

Focus on What We Can..., Not Why We Can't...

Whenever we bring together a group of people with different personalities, backgrounds, and organizational cultures into which they have been assimilated, we will find significant differences in outlooks. Of particular importance is one related to the concept of optimism. In many conversations, when innovative ideas arise, the discussions become challenging. We see each person select a place on the continuum between (1) figuring out how to implement that innovation and (2) identifying why that innovation won't work. In the public sector this tendency toward the latter is quite strong.

We need our mental health and addiction programs and their partnering organizations to develop a dominant culture of only focusing on how we can make such innovations or transformations work. We need to make it part of the intentional and explicit culture of the partnership. We need to build this concept into the painfully-written terms of reference for such collaborations, and then for that creative positivity to be actively supported, while constantly preventing the *yeah buts*. The representatives of partnering organizations or departments must explicitly discourage the members from ever focusing on the '*yeah but we can't do that because....*'. We can't allow people to identify a barrier unless they are also identifying a way to fix it or get around it. This kind of collective and creative optimism will facilitate innovation and real change.

Actions for system managers and leaders:

Promote optimistic, solution-oriented thinking and conversations among the partners, and explicitly discourage simple identification of reasons something cannot be done.

CHAPTER 11

TREATING THE 'WHOLE' CLIENT –
INTEGRATION OF ADDICTION SERVICES
AND MENTAL HEALTH SERVICES

To achieve good, client-centered service, there is a need for a fairly deep level of functional integration of these two formerly-separate program areas. As noted elsewhere in the book, people want and need to be treated as a whole, not as a collection of separate parts. These fields have evolved in relative isolation. Not only does our history include the mind and the body being seen and treated as independent of one another, but, even within the psychological/mental component, we have historically kept addictions separate from other kinds of closely-related struggles. This historical fact, and its somewhat illogical nature, has led over the years to much discussion about the need to integrate the programs providing addiction services and those providing mental health services.

These discussions go back well into the 1990s. However, during those early years the idea didn't get much traction for a few key reasons. First and foremost was reciprocal stigma. People with addictions commonly saw those other people as being *mentally ill*, which they themselves were not, in their opinions. Also, many people with mental illnesses saw those *addicts* as having bad decision-making and willpower problems (reminiscent of some of the paradigms from early days, like the moral model).

Even between staff there is a history of reciprocal stigma. The addictions staff saw the mental health folks as too restrictive in whom they would help, too pathology-oriented, and too strictly-governed by a medical model. This was seen as being so extreme that it failed to recognize all the other contextual factors in a person's life that contribute to his illness or wellness. Mental health staff saw the addictions staff as being less qualified, too open and loose regarding when and how they accepted clients into treatment, and generally having an easier job (because they considered addiction treatment to be a lower level of specialty and intensity, therapeutically speaking). After all, in their opinions, the addictions staff were just trying to talk people into getting more willpower. Stigma and its cousins *stereotype*, *prejudice*, and *discrimination* were all alive and well in both of these fields, among staff and clients.

The other key reason for resistance to such integration has been fear on the addictions side about being swallowed up by the larger and more dominant mental health programs. Despite the fact that the people in the programs would likely still continue to have employment and lots of work to do helping people with their issues, apprehension persisted. It arose out of a worry that the medical model on which mental health services were established would come to replace the more addiction-appropriate *biopsychosocial plus* model, described well by Marilyn Herie and Wayne Skinner (Herie & Skinner, 2014). This is a well-accepted, comprehensive model that recognizes the role of the biological, psychological, social, and spiritual components of a person's lived experience in relation to their addictions, and allows for all these components to be considered within treatment.

This apprehension was further compounded by a common belief that the medical model, by its very nature, was more expert-centered than client-centered (regardless of how client-centered the individual people delivering the services might have thought themselves to be). One final note was that wait times in the former mental health programs were generally much higher than in the former addiction services programs. In Nova Scotia, this difference was also reflected in the provincial standards, which essentially set the minimum target for what length of wait times were considered, by those running the system, to be acceptable (three months for mental health versus three weeks for addictions in Nova

Scotia provincial standards at that time). That tolerance for higher wait times in mental health was acilitated and enabled by the traditional, expert-centric, medical model described earlier. This created another reason for the smaller addictions program to be worried about being assimilated into the larger and less-responsive mental health system.

Over the past decade, we have seen many moves in the direction of structural integration. However, it is crucial to note that putting these two formerly-separate programs under a common structure or reporting to a common leadership position is not integration. It is merely putting both programs under a common leadership position. Remember, if your goal is client-centered service, in which people both *feel* and actually *are* treated as a whole persons, rather than a collection of separate psychological parts, more is needed. The system needs to function as one, all the way to the clinical level. It is not good enough merely to have separate programs that happen to report to the same person. The clinical level is the most important, from a client perspective.

There is an old saying in management that *form should follow function*. What that really means is that we should design a structure around the way we want a program or organization to operate. It is safe to say that this is a commonly-accepted principle. It makes sense intuitively that the most important thing is how an organization actually works. Therefore, if a structure can be created that is supportive of that work, it should be. However, as a social psychologist, I can say that there is more to it than that.

We know that people are constantly dividing themselves into groups that we consider to be *us*, and groups that we consider to be *them*. These are referred to in social psychology as *ingroup* and *outgroup*. This division is a perpetual part of the way we form our sense of connectedness and collective identity. For instance, if you are a woman, you may consider other women to be one of *us*, and consider men to be *them*. As a university faculty member, I consider faculty to be *us*, while I look at my students as being *them*. We identify ourselves as distinct collectives or groups based on virtually any meaningful and significant characteristic that we share with some people and not with others. We divide ourselves this way constantly, based on our jobs, professions, religion, country of origin, skin colour, financial status, education levels, and so on. It is a perpetual process, with virtually no limits, because it is solely based on our own perception of ourselves and our perceived similarities with and differences from others.

This has many implications and shows up in many different ways in our lives. It is strongly evident in partisan politics, fan loyalty to sports teams, and virtually anything of that competitive nature. It also shows itself in some very negative and destructive ways, such as international conflicts, and perceived or real inter-religious conflicts. Underlying all of these situations, and underlying many issues of stigma, oppression, segregation, prejudice, and discrimination is the basic perception of *difference* between *us* and *them*. We do not tend to experience any of these kinds of negative attitudes or behaviours toward people we consider to be *the same as us* or *one of us*. Instead, with those who are *one of us*, we tend to develop connection, relationship, and real or perceived cohesion.

So, let's apply this concept to the idea of integration between a mental health program and an addictions program. If our goal is simply organizational efficiency, then merely setting a common directorship accomplishes that goal to a very limited extent. However, if the management structure under that directorship is still segregated and distinct by addiction versus mental health program area, we have the us/them dynamics described above. If one person is managing part or all of the addiction program exclusively, and another is managing part or all of the mental health program exclusively, their focuses will naturally be on the component of the program for which they are individually responsible. After all, that is their job. Unfortunately, even if encouraged to think and work collaboratively, this will often be a struggle because they still have segregated and distinct responsibilities and, to some extent, will continue to think of the part they manage as *their* program.

Further to this, let's look at the client-service level. If a particular person is working in the addiction program, working with addiction colleagues, serving addiction clients, and reporting to the addiction manager, the resulting group identity that each member internalizes will take the form of addiction staff being *us* and mental health staff being *them*. This also runs the serious risk of addiction clients/issues being *ours* and mental health clients/issues being *theirs*, which brings us back to the splitting of the client into multiple parts. Likewise, the mental health staff will see themselves as *us* and the addiction staff as *them*, and will similarly perceive part of the clients' needs to be their responsibility and part not. Interestingly enough, this is the exact nature of our history. Because these fields evolved with that level of absolute independence from one another, these separate group identities and segregated components of treatment have been the norm.

So how do we get past this? Simply put, we need to take steps to create a singular sense of *us*. This requires a focus on several key things. They include name, structure, language, contact, and interdependence.

Factors Affecting Successful Integration

What's in a Name?

The official name of a program that gets marketed to the public is intended to tell all the citizens (i.e., current and potential clients) about its purpose and about the services it offers. It can either help people see themselves as potential users of the program, or not. The way this naming or formal *branding* is done can have an impact on the clients. In the past, we have had two separate programs with distinct names. The mental health services and programs have been most often known to the public as 'mental health', and the programs for addictions have been known by a greater variety of names because of programs being separate entities and identified under a specific name, such as Drug Dependency or Addiction Services (in Nova Scotia), Addiction Research Foundation (ARF) in Ontario, or the Alberta Alcohol and Drug Abuse Commission (AADAC).

In many areas, mental health services and addiction services have been brought together and integrated to various extents, ranging from full integration of services to a mere sharing of a single CEO, director, or other senior leader over the two programs that still clinically function separately from each other. When structurally merged, a single name is typically applied. For public clarity, that formal name needs to include terminology from both previous programs. The public needs to know it provides *mental health* services, and also that it provides *addiction* services. Otherwise, some clients are excluded by virtue of their not seeing their own health issues in the name of the program. If a car dealership sells Toyotas and Hondas, but is called Halifax Toyota, then we will not consider going there if we are looking for a Honda.

The two program areas have a dramatic difference in terms of size, budget, numbers of staff, and numbers of clients. In any such scenario, we need to take care to prevent the smaller one (services for people with addiction-related concerns) from being intentionally or unintentionally eliminated in practice or in name. If that were to happen, clients could stop seeing themselves as being welcome or as fitting in the service, which could reduce access by reducing self-identification and self-referral.

Here is where the risk exists. We abbreviate names and titles. We shorten terminology to the smallest version we can. We use Allie for girls named Allison, and Rob or Bob for boys named Robert. We use ED or ER for our emergency department, and DI for diagnostic imaging. We even disrespect some of our own citizens by using Newfoundland instead of the whole name of that Province, Newfoundland and Labrador. This is a natural tendency to be briefer, more efficient, or perhaps just lazy in our communication.

When we put *mental health* before *addictions* in the name, it very often becomes abbreviated to just *mental health*. Most readers have likely witnessed this many times. As long as mental health, the larger and more dominant program area, is at the beginning of the name, such abbreviation remains common. It is easy for people to drop the smaller, more specific terminology of *addictions*. This jeopardizes program identification and access by clients. People with addiction issues do not see themselves as needing to go to a program just referred to as mental health.

On the other hand, if a program were named *'addiction and mental health'*, the second half of the name would never be dropped in our tendency to abbreviate. It could not because of the relative size and dominance of the two program components. Clients, public, media, staff, etc., would always use the more-complete and inclusive name. They would never just call it 'addictions'. As a result, clients with addiction issues would always be able to see themselves in the name and know that is where they can get help, as would those experiencing mental illnesses. It is not a client-centered program if we do not anticipate the way a name will evolve and be used, and allow the name to facilitate the self-exclusion of potential clients.

Throughout the book, I have referred to this field informally as the mental health and addiction system, because the dominant psychiatric model being discussed as the subject of the book is primarily part of the former mental health programs. It therefore made sense to refer to it in this way here so the mental health component is most salient in the discussions. However, when naming a local program officially for public promotion, access, branding, advertising phone numbers and addresses, etc., it is important to consider the way the above-noted factors can directly impact on clients. Place 'addictions' first in the formal name, so both mental health and addiction clients know the program is there to help them.

Structure

As previously noted, the structure needs to support a single group-identity between the previously-separate mental health versus addictions staff perceptions. One way to achieve this is to create a structure that puts the two staff groups together at *every* level of the organization, especially in front-line management or supervision. This is the most important level of structural integration, despite the fact that many organizations have only focused on upper management. The upper levels are in fact the least important and least influential in terms of creating client-centered integration. This is mainly because they do not directly influence the ingroup-outgroup perceptions among clinical

TODD LEADER

staff. All management positions, to the greatest extent possible, need to have a scope of responsibility that crosses the historical gap between these program areas.

If a person is the front-line manager of all outpatient services (both addictions and mental health) in a particular geographic catchment area, she comes to view that portfolio as a single program, a single set of services, a single staff group, a single responsibility, and a single client population to be served. That means she will ignore the historical divide between the programs because it is truly irrelevant to her work. This frees her up to instinctively design systems and processes, and even further levels of structure, that are all-encompassing and directly support and promote the concept that we are *one* service.

As that front-line manager continues to build universal systems and processes, with an explicit disregard for the previous distinction between the two programs (conscious effort at first, gradually becoming instinctive or habitual), staff begin to identify themselves as a single group. They report to, and probably complain about, the same manager. When they have team meetings, their team is the combined group. When they have case conferences, *those other people* are there too. When they put together their working group to plan a program or event, it is again a mixed group. Throughout this process, what is happening is that people are reconstructing their definition of the *ingroup*, or of *us*. They begin to identify with one another as colleagues. They refer to the group as *we*, and no longer as *us* and *them*.

In reality, as we watch this happen, we see remarkable shifts in the way staff interact with one another and in the way they contribute to our goal of client-centered care. Other than a rare person, whose dogma or rigidity would never really allow them to make this conceptual shift, virtually all staff gladly (whether knowingly or unknowingly) reconstruct their group identity in this way.

Language

The language used by leaders in the program must be designed to intentionally support this concept of a singular, collective group-identity

206

across the program. This is not a complicated point, but it does involve breaking long-standing habits.

For instance, we may be used to referring to one group of people as the mental health staff and another as the addictions staff. We may be used to referring to one hallway in the building as the addictions hallway. We may also be in the habit of referring to some clients as mental health clients and some as addiction clients. This language needs to be eliminated. As long as we allow this terminology to continue to be used, it serves the purpose of cognitively maintaining the separate and distinct group identities that we are trying to eliminate. In order to create the single group identity (i.e., that sense of *we* versus *us* and *them*), we must consistently use inclusive terminology.

This is not a political-correctness point. It is a practical point. The single-group identity will not form effectively if people continue to refer to themselves and others by the old group names that represent separateness and distinctness. For instance, as long as people continue to think of themselves as the mental health staff or as seeing the mental health clients, they will not define themselves as part of an integrated addiction and mental health program.

Leadership teams must make concerted efforts to eliminate that old language from their own vocabularies. We need to catch ourselves referring to an *addictions* something or a *mental health* something, and shift it to the more-inclusive, single program name. We need to pay close attention during meetings to listen for those former ingroup-outgroup labels being used by staff, and then respectfully identify the slip so that it can be corrected. We need to watch the automatic signatures on people's emails to try to ensure that every staff member has changed the way they refer to themselves.

It must be acknowledged that there will sometimes be problems with infrastructure that inhibit this shift in language. If the *addiction clients* and the *mental health clients* are still being registered in separate client data systems, or kept in separate paper files, the language can't completely change. There will still be a need to identify clients by this

207

old terminology in order to manage the non-integrated client records. Even in such a case, the use of this language can at least be restricted to those specific situations.

As you can probably appreciate, this is not the kind of thing that is achieved as an overnight change. It is not merely a memo to instruct staff to do it differently. This is culture change. We need to work on this over quite some time. Even after years, we may still hear the occasional use of the older, divisive terminology, most likely from someone who has always been more attached to the past. Nonetheless, this is an important part of the effort to achieve the deep integration required for client-centered services. We can make all the structural changes we want, but if the people within the structures still refer to themselves and others in ways that indicate distinct sub-groups, integration and smooth collaboration will be limited because of that group identity.

Contact and Co-Location

There are many situations in which people in this field believe that co-locating staff is the secret to causing integration and collaborative work. This assumption is based on some very early research in social psychology known as the contact hypothesis. In its earliest and most simple form, it was based on the idea that if people from different groups spend time in close and frequent contact with one another, some of the typical ingroup and outgroup dynamics will dissipate. This work was investigated quite thoroughly during the time of desegregation of black and white students in American schools. As it turned out, this particular formulation of the idea was over-simplistic and ineffective.

Putting mental health and addiction staff together in one location will not, by itself, change those intergroup dynamics that keep them from collaborating as one team. That is not to say it is valueless. In fact, it does play a role. It can make a contribution if combined with other contextual factors. For instance, its influence can be enhanced if it provides opportunities for *social* interaction among members of the groups. This can be as simple as providing and encouraging the use of a common lunch room, or allowing for a small amount of time at team meetings for fun, ice-breaker kinds of activities that promote personal sharing, laughter, etc. (note I said a *small* amount because it also increases wait times). This can also be enhanced further by spreading the staff out so they are not clustered in their original groupings in particular hallways or physical spaces. Maintaining those older clusters would simply support the maintenance of separate group alliances and, more importantly, identities.

Interdependence

The extent to which intergroup contact can contribute to the formation of a single group identity is affected by the amount of dependence the members have on one another. In other words, the more a member of one group becomes dependent on a member of the other group to meet his own needs, the more he will start to see that other group member as part of the ingroup (i.e., one of *us*).

Some readers may recall from an introductory psychology or social psychology class in university, a reference to early research using a model known as the 'jigsaw classroom'. The essence of it is simple. In newly-integrated schools, racially-diverse learning groups were created in classrooms, in which each student was given only part of the total information they all needed to learn. Each one had a different portion of the information and was required to teach the rest of the group her own part of what they all had to learn. Therefore, no student could accomplish her own task (learning *all* the information for the test) without the help of *them* (the students previously thought of as part of that *other* group of people). The basic result was a reduction in some of the ingroup-outgroup thinking that had previously dominated and sustained racial segregation and prejudice.

We need to apply the same basic concept to people who think of themselves as mental health staff and those who think of themselves as addictions staff. If we create an environment in which members of the respective programs need one another in order to do their own jobs, it will contribute to progress. For instance, if there is a new group-therapy initiative to be developed, we could establish a team approach to developing it, and the team of perhaps two people would be inclusive of someone from each of the two previously-separate program areas. This makes those staff dependent on one another for their own success in the development and delivery of that service.

Another example lies in the assignment of clients. We need to begin gradually to schedule clients more flexibly and indiscriminately. A therapist who had previously worked in the addictions program might now be assigned a client who came for help with anxiety issues. A client with substance use issues might now be assigned to a person whose position had been within the previously-separate mental health program. Of course, that by itself does not create interdependence. However, when we have designed the system to be client-centered, it is not appropriate to have a client seen by multiple clinical staff unless there are complex specialty needs that can't be met in a less-intrusive way. In that context, each of the therapists being assigned clinical issues with which they have less experience has an increased requirement for consultation and reciprocal teaching and support. In other words, they need to consult and learn from their colleagues who have more experience in those issues. If they are discouraged from referring a client to each other, and instead expected to simply consult each other and do all the direct work with the client themselves, then they become interdependent. This reliance on each other for their own success and effectiveness will go a long way to creating a single program identity across the previously separate groups.

Actions for system managers and leaders:

1. Ensure that the formal, publicly-promoted name of the integrated program has the word 'addiction' coming first, to prevent an abbreviated version that leaves some clients excluded.

2. Ensure the program structure is integrated (combining *addiction* and *mental health* staff and programs) all the way down to the direct staff-supervisory level.

---

3. Attend closely to changing all use of language among staff that indicates or supports the separateness of the previous two programs, staff groups, or client populations.

4. Co-locate staff, and within a facility, ensure the workspaces/ offices of staff from both program areas are scattered and intermingled (not clustered or grouped by program area) throughout.

5. Ensure staff have space and opportunity for social interaction among the previously-separate groupings.

6. Create processes that require interdependence among staff, particularly across the previous lines of segregation (addictions versus mental health). In other words, make them need one another in order to be successful or effective in their own jobs.

Integration and Concurrent Disorders

Without a doubt, one of the primary motivators behind the idea of integrating mental health and addiction programs is improving the system's ability to do better work with people experiencing both mental illness and substance use issues. Let's consider how the integration work described above may impact on the care of people experiencing such co-occurring disorders or challenges.

First, reconsider the historical context. The primary reason we have generally not done a good job with these clients is that we perceived the programs, organizations, and professional groups to be separate. In that environment, concurrent disorder work has involved all of the awkwardness and inconvenience for the client described in previous sections.

Some have thought the solution to exist in the creation of standard screening and assessment processes, and specialized concurrent disorder services that are a distinct service stream, or staffed with a dedicated team. So, a program may have instituted a standardized tool that gathers information from every client during intake or first appointment to help flag those clients who have co-occurring disorders. That is problematic because it is reflective of the traditional medical/psychiatric model. It approaches the client from a position of presumed expertise, rather than from an assumption that the client knows what his needs are. It imposes an assessment process on every person, regardless of whether or not there is an indication of a need. It is contradictory to the idea of being the least intrusive we can be with clients. It harkens back to the days of putting every client through a standard assessment of everything **we** want to know, rather than respecting the client by asking him what he wants to tell us.

As noted, separate and dedicated 'concurrent disorder programs' or service streams have also been seen as an approach to treating clients with co-occurring disorders. This approach is flawed in a couple key ways. First and foremost, it assumes that the experience of co-occurring disorders is a rare event requiring a specialty focus. As our understanding of the data and the clients has evolved, it has become abundantly clear that this is false. Most people in the field now agree that a significant majority of all clients are experiencing a combination of mental health and addiction-related issues that are inextricably interwoven in their lives. Whether severe enough to call them *disorders* is irrelevant. With that established, we must conclude that concurrent disorder work does not really involve a separate specialty sub-group of clients, but rather needs to be a core function of the entire system. It is a common foundation of what our programs do. It is a core competency, not a specialty skill set. Therefore, a separate program or service stream would end up adopting most clients of the whole service, especially if inclusive of all those with co-occurring symptoms, issues, and problems, versus only *disorders.*

The second major flaw with the idea of a separate concurrent disorder program is that it reinforces stigma by creating yet another, distinct *type* of client. It says to the mental health client, and to the addictions client, and to the public, that this person is different from them. So much so that he requires a distinct and more complex specialty service. Remember, stigma relies on the perception of difference, as do prejudice and discrimination. Therefore, the more we do to carve off parts of our client population into smaller groupings of distinct (or different) kinds of clients or problems, the more we create or maintain stigma that is harmful to those clients. We need to normalize all levels and combinations of symptoms and disorders in these areas, as nothing more than health issues – like having hypertension and diabetes. We do that by avoiding the creation of new sub-types and new labels. We do that by avoiding the creation of new ingroup-outgroup distinctions that previously didn't exist.

Now, let's imagine that we have achieved the kind of real integration outlined in this chapter, to the point that staff no longer perceive themselves as two distinct groups. They are simply one group of co-workers who all deal with the full variety of individual or co-occurring symptoms or disorders presented by clients in areas of mental health and substance use. They have lunch together, team meetings together, and they depend on one another for expert assistance whenever a case requires it. Most importantly, they never use terms like *mental health* or *addictions* as identifiers when referring to clients, staff, or services.

In that kind of situation, is there any need for a standard one-size-fits-all screening or assessment for concurrent disorders? No, because *every* client's unique set of needs is discussed and examined to whatever extent the client wants. Is there any need for a separate stream of service for *concurrent disorder clients*? No, because most of that becomes instantly redundant and excessive when any staff member can be the care provider, with the assistance of other co-workers in the background.

In a fully-integrated program, beyond the superficiality of structure, and down to the level of clinical functioning and team identity, every client's needs are identified and addressed accordingly. Some will have one issue, and many will have more than one. Most of those who have multiple treatment issues will not need to be *referred* to someone else within the same program. They will not need to be scheduled to see two separate people and experience double the inconvenience, stress, loss of income, and other resulting hardships. They will simply come to appointments with the assigned therapist, who will do her job of treating that client's unique set of mental health and addiction issues. Any complications will be addressed automatically and efficiently between staff members in quick phone calls or office conversations.

In an integrated system, we can easily and naturally provide seamless, convenient, customized, client-centered treatment, regardless of the concurrent nature of their issues, and without the formality and awkwardness that came with the segregation of the past. We can achieve this, but only if we work to accomplish the psychosocial integration among the staff, using our understanding of intergroup relations. Structure alone won't get us there if perceived separateness still exists.

Actions for system managers and leaders:

To create a program that is responsive to co-occurring symptoms and illnesses, in a genuinely client-centered way, first place your focus on changing the intergroup relations and perceptions among the previously-separate staff groups. Concurrent disorder work will happen frequently and automatically as a result.

CHAPTER 12

DEVELOPING A CLIENT-CENTERED LEADERSHIP TEAM

Programs need managers and management teams. Their primary job and required skill set is to keep the train on the tracks, or to keep the program running according to the *status quo*. Programs also need leaders and leadership teams. Their role, regardless of position, is to determine where the new train tracks should go, and then get them built. Their job is to move the program in significantly different directions for the sake of improvement of the client experience. This is less about position and job title, and more about personality and skill set. If we want to be able to transform our systems from a medical and pathology-oriented paradigm, which are the long-standing, well-entrenched norm, we need *leaders*.

If we want to cause fundamental change to a program, we need a team that has a distinct set of characteristics. They need to be part oracle, so they can envision the future. They need to be natural optimists, so the vision they see is always positive and possible. They need to be like children looking forward to a trip to Disneyland, so they're always deeply excited about what is coming next. They need to be like Usain Bolt, able to sprint at any time to achieve short-term milestones. They need to have the unwavering perseverance of a marathon runner, who takes every leg of the race and every obstacle along the way as a thrilling personal challenge because of the cumulative payoff of achieving a good finish. They also need to be part rebel. That is, they need to recognize that change does not come from doing more of the same things we have always done, or doing those same things better. We need people, therefore, who, for client-centered reasons, instinctively want to push boundaries, challenge the *status quo*, challenge old traditional models, and be comfortable with a constant mix of being supported and being criticized.

In order to achieve a transformation to what clients and public would consider to be a client-centered system, the selection, development, and operation of a mental health and addictions leadership team needs to be guided by some key principles (described below). Without these, what will exist is a management team, not a leadership team. The train will stay on the tracks, and some of those tracks may be cleaned up and polished... but no new tracks will be built to take people to a better client experience.

We Are Client-Centered

Every member of the leadership team must fully understand, and *deeply* believe in, what it means for a *system* to be client-centered. The team must collectively understand that, no matter what they are discussing or struggling with, the *right* answer or the *right* decision is always the one that benefits the client the most, even if it is inconvenient for the staff, the leadership team, or them personally. They must have no loyalty to the *status quo*, the good old days, or the safety of stable predictability. Instead, they must be people who instinctively try to view the world, and the services, from the perspective of the client.

They must be people who have a strong sense of empathy because without it they cannot see the world from another person's viewpoint. They need to be people who notice injustices, inequities, and disadvantage because that will help them to see when our services cause those very things in our clients' experience. They must be individuals who recognize that we are not the experts whom the clients are lucky to get to see, but, rather, that it is we who are privileged to help the clients. If we follow tradition, we would select our leaders for administrative competence or clinical expertise, possibly without recognizing that neither quality is in itself sufficient nor even required to prepare one to lead such a change. If we want leadership teams that can transform our programs to become client-centered, we need people who already have client-centeredness as an instinct or even a personality characteristic.

Actions for system managers and leaders:

Select people to be part of a transformational leadership team based on their natural and deeply-passionate and empathic understanding of, and commitment to, a client-centered system. Ignore positions and titles and select the right *people*.

We Are One

The members of the leadership team in an *integrated* mental health and addiction program must continually recognize and remind themselves and one another that they are one team, responsible for one program. Regardless of the fact that there may be team members from various program settings or components, or with diverse backgrounds and histories, the team as a whole must function as a single, leadership entity. Their job is to work collectively to create a comprehensive, client-centered program. It is not like Parliament in which each member is supposed to represent and advocate for his/her own constituency or area of responsibility. It is a team that has a single responsibility to run a single program, for a single client... the taxpaying public. So, turf protection or us/them thinking cannot be allowed in the leadership team.

Furthermore, the team must continue to promote and reinforce the idea that the mental health and addiction program is not an island. It is merely one set of services that are part of a larger health care system/organization. Therefore, the job is to develop services that are integrated with all the components of health care, outside of their own program.

As described at length earlier, this sense of oneness, and single, organizational- and program-identity, is a critical piece of transformation.

The leadership team must be the ambassadors and messengers who continuously promote that cognitive shift.

Actions for system managers and leaders:

Ensure the leadership team actively, passionately, and consistently internalizes and promotes the single-group identity described at length in the previous chapter.

We *Fight* to Be Effective Rather Than Right

As a social psychologist, I am never surprised, yet always disturbed, by the extent to which people in the workplace are averse to disagreement, dissent, and debate. So, why is this a problem? It does make sense that we would want people to get along in the workplace. Clearly, we should try to achieve a peaceful work environment for staff. The problem with the absence of disagreement is the previously-described phenomenon of *groupthink*, which is known to lead to bad decision-making by groups. This is not necessarily a conscious decision to engage in groupthink. There may be other dynamics at play that are subtle but powerful.

To start with, many of us are taught as children that we should not fight with others. In reality, if you look closely at what children are doing when they are told that, often it is merely arguing and disagreeing about something. This discouragement of arguing becomes even stronger when adults or authority figures come into play. We advocate even more fervently with our children not to disagree with their parents, teachers, and other authority figures. They may not be required to agree, but they are forbidden from disagreeing, even if it is done respectfully. That only leaves one option, which is silent acceptance or apathy regarding something you don't agree with.

Let's transition into the workplace. We have been taught, and have come to believe at least to some extent, that disagreeing and arguing are undesirable behaviors. Therefore, we try our best not to do so. Bring the boss into the room at the same time, and our aversion to disagreement is strengthened because she is an authority figure. Now, let's add another dynamic to that. Many people in management and leadership positions are not open to dissonance, or to the insinuation that they might be wrong. Therefore, in such workplaces employees' previously-learned avoidance of argumentation is reinforced by the established workplace culture under that authoritarian leadership style.

The question we all need to ask ourselves as leaders is whether we would rather be right or be effective. Hopefully, both of these can occur together once in a while, but it is common to see a leader's need for one of these undermine her ability to achieve the other. They are often incompatible. For instance, have you ever known someone in a leadership position who did not like to be challenged or disagreed with, or was not open to debate? Perhaps someone who would react either emotionally or dismissively to the suggestion that her ideas or plans were not actually the best way. If you have, you have likely observed that this person struggled to achieve any significant change or to lead a program to any truly-remarkable accomplishments. On the other hand, have you known someone who was intolerant of settling for mediocrity in the departments or organizations she led? A person whose compulsion to be effective as a leader of change, and to help the organization achieve great positive results, would lead her to be willing to change any decision or plan in order to get there. This is a person who wants to be effective more than she wants to be right.

Many of us have witnessed both extremes, as well as seeing many people at other points on the continuum. One of the key differences in these two styles is that one discourages disagreement, while the other welcomes or even *insists* on it. Leadership teams must create an environment in which the members regularly engage in passionate disagreement. It needs to be an *intentional* culture of debate. If someone has a difference of opinion from what is being discussed at a meeting and does not share it, that should be frowned upon.

When a leader creates this kind of debate-oriented culture in her team, it pretty much guarantees two things. First, it ensures that the mental health and addiction program has 100% of the best thinking of every person on the leadership team, contributing to the best decisions for the clients. Second, it guarantees that every member, including the leader, is often wrong, or at least is not the one whose idea is supported and determined to be the best. With this type of approach, only the best ideas win, and it does not discriminate based on title, experience, or the extent to which a person talks the most or the loudest. It relies solely on analysis of what is best for clients.

Creating this environment allows a mental health and addiction leadership team to focus exclusively on being effective at creating the most client-centered service possible. No matter what any person might prefer personally or might believe to be the best decision, each other person there has one job and that is to make sure the team ends up making the right decisions for the right reasons. The moral and pragmatic compass that this style creates should not be underestimated. It is incredibly powerful at helping a program achieve truly-transformative change.

> **Actions for system managers and leaders**:
>
> Create and insist on active and passionate debate and disagreement within the leadership team. This must be driven by, and exclusively focused on, identifying only the best and most effective client-centered decisions.

We Empower Each Other to Lead

If we want a leadership team to thrive and to bring about transformative change, its members need to have the freedom and encouragement to do so. This is a very straightforward concept for those who are already inclined in this direction, and an elusive and threatening concept for those not. The essence of it is that if we want to achieve change in such a complex system as mental health and addictions, or any aspect of health care for that matter, we can't do it alone or in an autocracy. We need to nurture the leaders. These leaders then need to have explicit freedom to create.

They need to know that their job is to make decisions, to make changes, to take risks by trying things a new way, and to challenge the way things were done in the good old days (or are done at present). They need to know that they can do all of this, and even if things turn out badly, they are safe because the leader they report to (their boss) supports them in that empowered, creative, risk-taking leadership. They need to know that their superiors will take full responsibility for anything that they try *for the right reasons*, even if it does not work out. They need to be decision-makers and change-agents, not people who need to check all such decisions and actions with someone else first. Coordination of efforts is one thing. Centralized control of decision-making and approvals is another. Without explicitly providing that true empowerment, which is comprised of the real and perceived freedom, power, ability, and support to bring about change, then we are not creating and nurturing leaders. We are simply managing managers.

Nurturing real leadership skills, frequently contrasted with management skills for obvious reasons, is one of the most important and effective tools in facilitating system transformation. The members of a leadership team must be given the following explicit messages through the words and actions of their program leader:

(1) They can make decisions any time about anything if the decision is in support of a more client-centered service.

(2) For major changes that intersect with other components of the overall program, they should bring it to the leadership team for debate and coordination.

(3) Case by case, day by day, as situations arise the leaders have the full right to handle and respond to problems, even if it means making exceptions to standard processes, or spending reasonable amounts of money.

(4) As noted above, the leaders must know, without *any* doubt, that if any decision or action they take for the right reasons (client-centered service) were to turn out badly, the person they report to would take full responsibility and they would never be negatively affected by such a situation. A good leader should have no problem making such

a commitment because a good leader believes in the normality and inevitability of making mistakes in the process of system transformation. New and innovative reform of an archaic system cannot come without trying things that have never been tried before. Inevitably, this must and does lead to mistakes. Those are not a problem, but a learning opportunity.

(5) The final thing that the members of a program's leadership team must understand clearly is that they can ask for and expect to receive the full support (input, ideas, debate, challenge, disagreement, etc.) of any of the other leadership team members, including the person they report to, at anytime, in order to achieve the best client-centered decision. This should function with a primary focus on challenging and questioning, which is the best way to support each other at being effective rather than right.

This same approach applies to the way the leadership team works with staff. Staff also need to be empowered to be creative, to make judgements and decisions when they need to be made, and to make exceptions to rules and procedures, if it is what is best for the client at the time.

Taking this approach, a mental health and addiction program will create an environment of creativity for its leadership team, and its staff – an environment of pure innovation that does not recognize restrictions and limitations. This is a culture of quality in its truest sense, focused entirely on doing the right things for the right reasons. This needs to be a deeply-principled group of people who will not compromise and accept anything short of excellence. They must know that they have the right, the freedom, and the obligation to think outside the box because that is where leadership truly exists.

Actions for system managers and leaders:

Explicitly empower the leadership team members, and the staff, to make decisions, be innovative, make exceptions to standard processes, and be creative in taking risks, as long as it is for client-centered purposes.

If Things Aren't Changing, We're Not Leading

The concepts of motion and transformation are intrinsic to the root of the word 'lead'. One of the items we may use to take a dog from one place to another is a lead. When we establish a project, we assign a lead, which is the person who will *move* the project forward. In a race, the person, car, or perhaps horse that is *moving* the fastest is in the lead. Leadership requires movement and change. If things are staying the same and not moving forward in significant ways, then leadership is not happening. Management might be, but leadership is not.

This is much more prevalent in the public sector than the private sector because, in business, failing to constantly change and adapt means you don't make a profit or don't get paid. In the public sector, change is sometimes frowned upon because it creates political uncertainty for governing parties. They may not always be sure how the changes will be perceived by the voting public. So, although it may be explicitly endorsed, making systems move and change is often implicitly inhibited.

We have all known people who, while in a leadership position, stood still. They did not make things move or change. Many of us have also seen people in leadership positions who engage in tweaking and adjusting things, but never fundamentally change the underlying flaws in the system. That's really just like changing the artwork on the walls in the same room you have been in all along. It's cosmetic. It's optics. There are still others who may manage a fundamental change, but only when given a roadmap. Many people in public-sector leadership have demonstrated the ability to take someone else's vision and methodology and merely implement it. That is clearly a sign of good management because following such an implementation process requires a person to be good with details, and able to put his head down and keep going step by step following instructions until complete. But, that is not leading, it is following.

It is the same as the distinction between a chef and a cook. If a chef creates a new and unique recipe, and a cook uses it and makes that meal, which one is *leading*? Clearly, it is the one who identified the vision for the meal and the direction for how to achieve it. The person doing the cooking is technically following and the chef is leading.

In program transformation, the same difference exists. Leadership is about creating program directions, principles, values, and a culture that supports creative, flexible, empowered, ongoing improvement. Following an implementation plan for a pre-packaged program someone else created is good management. We need both in our mental health and addiction programs, but our system will never be transformed by management. It will require people who are leaders to see a new direction.

Leadership is about identifying the need (out of a constant intolerance for imperfection in a system), identifying the vision, then inspiring and supporting people to collectively cut a new path toward that vision regardless of the obstacles. As stated earlier, if we truly want to transform the system, we need people with no attachment to history, and who never quote the good old days. We need people who are naturally and incessantly optimistic. These are people who never identify barriers or reasons why we can't move forward unless they are simultaneously identifying the path around those barriers. They do not see obstacles, but, rather, only turns we need to take in the road. We need people who are creative and regularly express ideas that no one has had before, and that sound odd, unrealistic, or out of place in the current context. We need the kind of people who might even make you worry about them running too fast for the system, and pushing change prematurely. We can help such natural leaders to slow down, but it is much harder to teach natural followers to lead.

To achieve the kind of transformation of paradigms and systems described in this book, programs need to develop a leadership team made up of *change-leaders*. If a program can assemble a team comprised of several people of this kind, no level of transformation will be impossible. However, it is very important to note that the first step is not the act of assembling the people who are already in the leadership positions, to form this team. The first step is to fill the leadership positions (regardless of whether formal, informal, union, management, etc.) with these kinds of people (leaders), and then put them in a room together and start visioning. Once that starts, keep reinforcing the idea that if things aren't changing, you're not leading. Simply managing or tweaking the existing system will not change the client experience. Nor will simply doing more of what has always been done, or doing it better. Regardless of anyone's attachment to traditional approaches, remember, *it's not about us.*

Actions for system managers and leaders:

Select your team members for their intolerance of imperfection and the status quo. Select people, regardless of their position, who crave real change.

We Do More *Doing* Than *Planning*

One of the other variables we need to pay attention to is the distinction between planners and doers, and between planning and doing. This distinction plays out like a child's seesaw. The more of one we do, the less of the other we do. The more we plan the less we do, and the more we do the less we plan. As noted earlier in the book, the public sector is often perceived by its funders (tax-paying public) as being more focused on the planning side than the doing. Whether that is a justified perception or not depends on who the leaders are in any given department, program, or organization.

Some people in leadership roles will want to collect and analyze every bit of data and information available, try to create the perfect plan to achieve a desired improvement, and try to anticipate everything that could go wrong so that mitigations can be developed. Those sitting on the other end of the seesaw will look at an issue and make impulsive decisions to act on it, with little to no consideration of available information, or potential obstacles or barriers., and so on. Clearly neither of these extremes is ideal. But, where is the best place on the see-saw for a transformational leadership team in a mental health and addiction program at this point in time? It would be too easy to simply say they should be in the middle with a good balance of both. Isn't that just like picking a medium popcorn at the movie theatre because you can't decide between a small and a large? There is a better answer.

Given the historical and widespread perception of the public sector as planning and not doing, it may be argued that we need to move more significantly in the direction of action. This is not to say we should eliminate planning. Instead, it is suggesting that we do the *minimum* amount of planning necessary to be able to identify and take the first actions. We need to stop trying to foresee every step and obstacle on the path. That is impossible. We need people leading who have the courage to begin cutting a new path and moving in the direction of the vision, without knowing everything they are going to come across along the way.

That means being prepared for *unexpected* challenges, and that also means these leaders need to be comfortable making mistakes, changing a decision, and moving on. So, where should a mental health and addiction leadership team be sitting on the seesaw? They should be on the action side of the fulcrum. If not, we may see even more decades of the kind of tiny, incremental adjustments that are safe and foreseeable in the planning, but do not actually transform the fundamental paradigm of the system or transform the client experience.

> **Actions for system managers and leaders:**
>
> Select your leaders based on their being doers more than planners.

We Don't Tolerate Non-Client-Centered Behaviour

The leadership team of a mental health and addiction program that wants to transform to a client-centered paradigm needs to work toward and arrive at a zero tolerance approach to non-client-centered behaviour among staff. Initially, in trying to move this transformation forward, the primary job is consistent and clear communication of what this change means at a behavioural and process level. This is not meant to be a patronizing statement. It is simply meant to reinforce the earlier point that staff have been working inside a medical model and culture that is long-standing, entrenched, and is in fact the only *normal way of doing things* that many of those currently in the system have ever known. As a result, the psychiatric, pathology-oriented paradigm is so strong and compelling that people will have a hard time being willing, or sometimes being able, to understand and accept the change. An expert-driven program is all we know.

Over the first several months of the transformation, the leadership team must regularly introduce the concept of a client-centered system, as distinct from client-centered therapy, and as distinct from an individual staff member being compassionate, empathic, and caring about the clients. This differentiation is absolutely vital to state, restate, explain, re-explain, and demonstrate through examples repeatedly. The impact of not doing so is that staff will perceive the change as being somehow a criticism of them individually, and a suggestion that, up to this point, they have not been client-centered. Psychiatrists will perceive it as a criticism of their very profession, which it clearly is not. In this book, I have repeatedly stated that such an implication is not part of the message. Good, compassionate staff do good, compassionate work on a daily basis. Psychiatrists provide excellent care every day for those in need of that level and type of intervention. On the other hand, the system that structures the client experience on the way to and from those interactions with clinicians is the primary focus of this proposed transformation.

Nevertheless, because staff have learned a traditional way of doing things in these programs, based on that expert-driven, medical model, there will be a need for behavioural norms to change. This is the part that must be described, in concrete terms, so that staff understand what is expected of them in the new approach. If not described in behavioural terms, staff will be left to use their own interpretation, and ambiguity and inconsistency will reign. For example, we cannot simply say things like 'we will respect the clients', or 'we will respect the client's time'. Those statements can mean absolutely anything, and therefore can mean absolutely nothing. They will not necessarily mean we will offer evening or weekend appointments to fit the client's life, or that we will reduce the amount of meeting time to allow better access to clinician appointments. Concrete descriptions of how such values and principles are to be operationalized at the behavioural level are needed.

Ambiguity of terminology is well known to fail to produce behavioural change. That is why the alcohol industry, for example, created and uses the term 'drink responsibly'. It means something different to every person, and every person can feel comfortable, within her own interpretation of it, that she is drinking responsibly. It has no effect on behaviour (types or amounts of alcohol consumption) because of its openness to subjective interpretation (which is why Big Alcohol uses it of course). Changing our system to being client-centered will require that we avoid that kind of ambiguity and use concrete statements of behaviour, like those used throughout this book to describe what needs to actually be *done*.

After all of the work getting staff to the point of recognizing the focus is on system change, not staff-blaming, and having them understand the behavioural implications of the transformation to this paradigm, accountability for individual-level behaviour must then be established. Again, to be repetitive because of the importance of the message, almost all staff in any mental health and addiction program will understand, accept, and adapt to this change. This section about accountability is not about them. It is about the exceptions. It is about the very few who – because of attachment to the past, dogmatic or self-serving loyalty to the expert-based, medical model, or general lack of adaptive and coping skills – will not change.

In those rare cases, the behaviour must be addressed consistently and progressively right up to whatever level of formal intervention is needed to either change the behaviour or remove the employee. In the public sector, which is virtually all unionized, there is a common aversion to taking on those performance-management and discipline cases. Managers often operate with a fear of grievances because they take a lot of time, and can frequently be turned around by the employee as an attack on the manager for his having addressed the behaviour. If we want to transform our system, that hesitancy needs to stop. The senior leaders need to empower managers to be intolerant of inappropriate (especially non-client-centered) behaviour, and to address it formally to whatever extent may be required.

It is very common in such a workplace for the majority of staff also to want that small minority to be held accountable, but they will not often come forward to complain or testify against co-workers on the record. So, it does fall to the managers.

Rest assured that if a manager operates according to the principles of client-centeredness described in this book, coupled with the basic principles of respectful workplace behaviour, she will be respected by the majority. She will also likely be disliked and treated aggressively by the minority who want to keep things their way. If she takes on the bad behaviour and forces it to change or for it to be pushed out, the majority will have even greater respect for her as a manager. They will, in fact, see her as a leader for having the courage to do what is right for the clients and for the employees in the workplace, despite making her unpopular among those she disciplined.

If the leadership team tolerates inappropriate and non-client-centered behaviour, the transformation will not move forward very effectively. It has a great risk of stalling because the message being sent is one of individual discretion. People see one employee continuing to do things the old way, perhaps over-assessing things that are not relevant to the client, and it tells them that client-led conversation is optional, not required. Well, we have had that for decades. Many such things have always been optional. Every individual behaviour in this book is optional to some extent, and is practiced inconsistently across most programs, based on each individual employee's priorities and values. The point to the client-centered transformation described here is to make it all consistent, reliable, and normal, regardless of who the staff members are, but for it to be based on principles that also allow it to adapt to client exceptions. That is what a paradigm shift for the system really is.

> **Actions for system managers and leaders:**
>
> Assertively manage and address non-client-centered behaviour by staff, using formal processes, in order to demonstrate a commitment to the paradigm shift and to improving the client experience.

> **Actions for clients, supporters, and advocates:**
>
> If you are ever treated disrespectfully by a mental health and addiction staff person, in a way that violates the kinds of client-centered principles described here, formally report that to the manager. Managers have a hard time stopping such behaviour if they have no formal complaint about it.

We Listen to Clients

Clients make their views known to the public mental health and addiction programs on a regular basis. Some do so through written feedback. Some file formal complaints. Some send in compliments through various mechanisms. Some even make their experience known through mass media and public interviews. In any case, and regardless of the reason or the positive or negative nature of the feedback, this is incredibly valuable information. It is in fact the most important kind. If we believe that our job is to create and offer services that put the client first, then we must respect and welcome their views.

When a client goes to the media, or goes directly to a program or organization with comments, what he is providing is the one thing we cannot actually know and understand without his direct input. He is providing his subjective, individual experience of our services. He is telling us how the steps in our process have either helped or harmed his ability to gain access. He is explaining how his interactions with our people, facilities, and paperwork have either helped or hindered his recovery. He is telling us the components of the program that are either client-centered or not. That information is exactly what is needed.

Our various professionals in the system have great expertise in clinical areas, including the effectiveness of diagnosis and treatment methods for all types of mental illness and addictions. That is the great strength of the current psychiatric/medical model. The piece that is missing from that expertise is what it feels like to be a client going through the services we provide. What is missing is expertise about the client experience, because only the client has that. The leadership in our public mental health and addiction system must listen hard, and non-defensively, when clients speak, and then consistently and perpetually apply that unique insight to the system transformation. We must use what is said, in every complaint or other type of feedback, to improve the client experience, and hence, the client-centeredness of the program.

Actions for system managers and leaders:

Listen non-defensively, and genuinely take all client complaints and feedback as an opportunity to improve.

Actions for clients, supporters, and advocates:

Regularly provide feedback (positive and negative) to management of your local program so they can keep learning and improving.

We Hire the Right Skills for The Right Jobs

If we are successful, our systems will start to make a real move away from thinking about everything as an acute care, psychiatric kind of problem, and stop thinking of only ill people as our clients. Then, by necessity and intention, the system will start providing more service to all the other people along the continuum, or who have needs for lower-tier services. This will require us to rethink our approach to staffing.

Currently, we hire heavily in the areas of psychiatry, psychiatric nursing, clinical psychology, and clinical social work. In Nova Scotia, these make up the majority of all staff positions. In theory (although it varies from one post-secondary school to another), all of these folks are primarily trained to provide either medical or psychotherapeutic interventions for people experiencing addiction or mental health problems. That is great for the more-acute or intensive services at the higher tiers. As indicated earlier, such professions are not necessarily the best fit with the work that is needed at the lower tiers, or at the earlier end of the continuum. It is important that we consider best fit, so we do not over-serve or under-serve our clients.

This has become a focus across health care. We try not to have a doctor do what a registered nurse can do. We try not to have a registered nurse do what a licensed practical nurse can do. This approach ensures that each classification works to its full scope, making the work a better fit with the need, and making the most efficient use of all the resources by keeping each level free for what is necessary. If a doctor is doing duties that a RN can do, that is time taken away from patients who need a service that only a doctor can provide.

For people experiencing life challenges, or very early and mild difficulties with substance use, stress or anxiety, or depressive feelings, they likely do not require psychiatric intervention, and often will not require psychotherapy. That means they don't need a clinical psychologist or psychiatrist, for instance. They may need some level of supportive and skill-building counselling that helps them learn to monitor and manage these issues and feelings, and prevent progression if possible. If we want to serve them with the most appropriate resource, we would do so with someone specifically trained for that purpose. This might be a para-professional counsellor with a college diploma trained in exactly that level of supportive, skill-building, problem-solving counselling. Such background is an excellent fit with this earlier-intervention and lower-clinical-complexity work. Not only do they do great work with the clients because of the fit between need and skill set, but they also allow the public resources to be used in the most efficient way (the former being the main purpose and the latter being a bonus).

Perhaps the greatest barrier to moving in this direction is professional elitism, which prevents this kind of goodness-of-fit and efficient use of resources. The phenomenon manifests itself as a concern about competency. We will hear people regularly disparage the professions they believe are less competent than their own. There is a perceived but unspoken hierarchy that starts with psychiatrists and moves *downward* to clinical psychologists, clinical social workers, registered counselling therapists, then paraprofessional counsellors.

In addition, conversations consistently call for all staff to be part of a legally-regulated profession. This is stated as being an issue of liability, of having someone accountable to an organization other than just the employer. But, if we hire for competencies, and if we manage our staff effectively, these are not issues that should over-ride providing the right kind of service for the needs of the clients, and using our taxpayers' dollars appropriately. These are not compelling arguments against hiring the kinds of staff required for the great many clients in need of lower-tier, prevention and early-intervention services. Professional elitism and a perceived but not-significant need for external accountability are not higher *priorities* than the needs of the client.

The final point in relation to hiring the right people for the right jobs is that we need to start hiring leaders for their leadership competencies. In health care broadly, we have a tendency to hire based on clinical skills and experience. The best nurse gets the job of the unit manager. The best clinician becomes the supervisor. We have an assumption that greater clinical expertise translates to leadership skill. That is absurd. That is like hiring the best electrician to fix your toilet. An abundance of one skill set does not equate to having a completely separate skill set. So, when we hire managers, we need to hire them because they are good managers, not good clinicians or nurses. When we hire leaders, we need to hire them because they are good leaders, not because they are good managers. To transform the system, we need to hire the right skill sets for the right jobs.

> **Actions for system managers and leaders**:
>
> Break tradition. Become aware of any of your own biases, and then begin to hire counsellors for counselling, and therapists for therapy. Hire managers to manage and leaders to lead.

> **Actions for clients, supporters, and advocates**:
>
> Advocate for funding to be used more efficiently by hiring counsellors to counsel and only hiring therapists or psychiatrists if it is to provide therapy or psychiatric intervention. It will improve access to early intervention support.

We Inspire with Vision, Not Indicators

We need a team that can see the future, a bright future, and can always convey that to others. The team members need to have an ability to describe a client-centered approach to system design, and do it in a way that people get excited and feel inspired to achieve that vision. Our history of trying to lead with indicators needs to come to an end, or be put in its place within management rather than leadership.

An effective leader and leadership team don't rely on such approaches to motivate staff and partners. Leadership requires emotional investment in sparking passion in people. Anyone can share numbers and facts, and make rational arguments about why something needs to change. However, that will only work for a small number of people, and won't work well. People need to be *inspired* to lead and participate in this change. They need to *feel* it. They need to get excited and feel passion for the vision of people having better access, being made to feel happy and satisfied, being made to feel welcome, safe, and respected. They need to be driven by the vision of people being made to feel relief that the right services are there to help, no matter the level or type of concern they have, and being made to feel like they are not alone. The leaders must be able to get excited themselves about such things and, more importantly, must have the ability to inspire others with such a vision.

Actions for system managers and leaders:

Select your leaders based on their ability to inspire people with vision and passion, and continue to help them further develop that skill and that way of being.

Actions for clients, supporters, and advocates:

Those among you who have this ability to inspire people to see and strive for a vision, and to feel passionate commitment to it, please use those skills. Inspire the public, the media, the government, the mental health and addiction staff and management, at every chance you get. The more visionary leaders we have inspiring this client-centered paradigm shift, the sooner we will make progress toward the vision. Talk about this, and get people excited about achieving it.

CHAPTER 13

THE MAKING OF CLIENT-CENTERED
SERVICES; CASE EXAMPLES

The process of transforming to a client-centered system has no limits within a mental health and addiction program. There is no such thing as a service, a process, a form, a policy, a physical structure, a staffing decision, etc., that can remain unexamined or is immune to improvement in this regard. As we took the program of South Shore Health through the transformation, we constantly found ways to challenge the historical processes and tendencies through which the system unknowingly treated clients as a lower priority than something or someone else.

This chapter provides a brief description of real programs that were either created or changed to be more client-centered, following the principles and approaches articulated in this book. To be clear, these are not meant to be examples of perfection or of best practice. They are meant to be examples of how we used the client-centered perspective to analyze each and every component of service, and then made attempts to improve them. They are merely examples of the kinds of developments and changes that can take place if we start to apply this client-centered paradigm to replace the current pathology-oriented, system – and expert-centered model.

Of course, this book does not allow for a lot of details, but does highlight some of the core aspects and most fundamental processes. It is important to note that these kinds of initiatives were the primary cause of dramatically-improved access and client experience in the south shore of Nova Scotia.

Example 1 – School-based Services for Adolescents

This first program example is responsible for adolescent wait times dropping from five months to same-day/same-week access (best wait times in Nova Scotia), and these changes have been sustained for several years. This particular program was the result of an incredibly advanced partnership between the South Shore Regional School Board and the former South Shore Health (now part of the Nova Scotia Health Authority).

Co-leadership and Co-management
between Health and Education

There are many jurisdictions in which joint committees exist between the health and education systems. However, in this case, our group was created entirely in accordance with the earlier section on collaborative partnerships. The Health and Learning Committee was a joint committee that directly and literally co-managed all collaborative initiatives between the two sectors.

This committee included only decision-makers (directors, managers, coordinators), so there was never a need to leave a decision hanging, pending someone else's approval. It was solely focused on what was best for the students, regardless of the work, money, inconvenience, or complication that it might cause to the two organizations. It was solely focused on decisions and actions, not information-sharing. If information was not meant to create a decision or action, then it was not shared there. The committee had a well-developed and intentional culture of frank discussion and debate, again focused only on determining what was best for students. It also had a well-developed and intentional culture of self-critical reflection, such that each member came to the table looking to improve his/her own contribution to the programs and processes, not the other's.

The committee recognized that health and education are not independent of one another. Education is a determinant of health, and health (especially mental health, addictions, and sexual health) is a determinant of a person's success in school. It had a well-developed and intentional culture of trust. The partners knew that they were all there for only one reason, and that was to constantly improve the health and the education of students. As part of that sense of trust, the trouble-shooting of problems that arose became an easy process.

The interagency collaboration between the school board and the health authority was constructed exactly according to all the criteria described in the earlier chapter on partnerships and interagency collaboration. Every aspect of that partnership matched this approach perfectly. Suffice to say that this relationship became the envy of both health and education across many areas of Nova Scotia, where the same depth of the relationship was never fully achieved. In fact people from other areas of Canada even visited to explore this model.

All members of the Health and Learning Committee maintained a constant and deeply-held understanding of the simple idea that *it's not about us.*

Program Background and Development

The vision was clear. It was March of 2012. By September, we were going to be in every middle school and every high school, delivering the most client-centered services possible for adolescents in our area. Identifying the specific needs was not a complex research question. Our school board partners already knew from years of watching and listening to their students. The three big issues for which they needed support were mental health, substance use, and sexual health. That fact informed our very first client-centered decision for this service. We were a program mandated to deal with mental health and addiction. If we had thought of our program as an independent entity, and if we thought rigidly of our formal mandate as being the priority (above the needs of the clients/students), then we would likely have dismissed sexual health as someone else's responsibility. If we had done that, we would have implicitly been deciding that clients' needs should fit our program structure, rather than our program making services fit clients' needs. In other words, we had the choice to be program-centered or client-centered. We chose to focus on the fact that *it's not about us*. It's about the client.

Coming at this from the perspective that we were merely one part of a single, client-centered health authority, we were not trapped by that program-centric thinking. We were able to avoid the historical tunnel vision that had kept the mental health program from ever being properly integrated into the school system. It had also kept both the mental health program and the addiction services program from ever being properly integrated (as opposed to co-located) with each other, or with related components of the health system, such as emergency departments or primary health care. In the past, all these pieces had functioned as if they were islands.

Fortunately, through the majority of the program-development phase for these school-based services, we had highly-skilled, visionary leaders in South Shore Health. They promoted true collaboration and integration as described throughout this book. They promoted innovation and risk-taking. They certainly understood that if we wanted to create a client-centered system, we would need to be prepared to bring down the walls between programs and organizations, to expand our mandate flexibly, and to customize our work in meeting the needs of the people we serve.

As a result, we did not have any problem including sexual health among the issues that our mental health and addiction counselling staff would support in the schools. It would just make no sense for a health authority to send in counselling staff to deal with mental health and addiction issues, and not also be prepared to have supportive and educational conversations about sexual health. This would have been illogical partly because it would not be client-centered, and also because it would be inefficient to have an additional person or department providing that sexual health service when we were already engaging and building trusting relationships for such conversations. If the needs of the adolescents were for support with mental health, substance use, and sexual health, then that was what we should and would provide. Staying within our traditional program structures and functions, frankly, was not important enough when compared to meeting the three top needs of our adolescent clients. *It's not about us.*

With the first hurdle over, and the client-centered approach winning out, we were ready to start building. The structure was not really complex. Most adolescents have some need for only low-intensity support and counselling, a smaller number need therapy, and even fewer need high-intensity, specialist intervention (psychiatry). So, we developed a tiered system that would be heavy on the individual-level education and early-intervention, supportive counselling.

This would represent a significant change from the way the former *mental health* program had worked in the past. While we did have full-time, paraprofessional, addiction counsellors in the schools for over 20 years in this catchment area, the involvement of the mental health program during that time was for psychotherapeutic intervention only (in accordance with the dominant paradigm). The work was also not built into the infrastructure of the schools. Therapists would go to schools to see clients on an as-required basis, and only those in need of intensive services (not those who were well, but needing support and help to stay that way). Nonetheless, this first level of paraprofessional counselling service was to be the foundation, the entry point, and the most-frequently needed and used part of the program.

Most of the staffing of this school-based service was achieved by reassigning existing staff members to work in the schools instead of in our centralized office (There was one exception that 2.5 therapists were provided through a new office. There was one exception that 2.5 therapists were provided through a new provincial initiative at that same time, called Schools Plus, which became another component of our great collaborative partnership between the health and education systems). This movement of our staff into the schools was initially a concern for some who thought it would diminish capacity. They worried that taking staff out of our main clinic and placing them in the schools would make the workload at the clinic unmanageable.

This concern about moving staff out of a centralized clinic was previously addressed in some detail in the chapter on early intervention. To briefly recap, there are three key factors to remember. First, it is the right thing to do. We can't claim to be client-centered, and claim to want to improve access, and then refuse to bring services out to the people being served. Decentralization of services is client-centered. Second, the staff moving out to the schools would still be seeing clients, but would merely be doing so in a *different location*. Third, and finally, the more we could provide this briefer, early-intervention support for youth who were not yet experiencing any clinical disorders, the fewer adolescents would require the intensive and time-consuming, therapeutic interventions. While this might increase uptake of early intervention counselling, it would also reduce demand for therapy. We would be making our services proportionately match the needs of our client, the public.

This was a major departure from the medical model that had dominated the mental health field for decades. Under that traditional model, as described earlier, the idea of supporting and counselling people who are not ill, but need help to stay well, would not have been in scope. If we wanted to help support healthy adolescents to stay healthy, we would need people with a different perspective and a different skill set. We needed people who were skilled at relating to young people informally, teaching life skills, coaching youth on life decisions, mentoring adolescents, motivating and empowering them, and helping them navigate the stresses and emotional ups and downs of normal life. For this level of support, we would need people who were **not** trained specifically to look for, identify, and diagnose illness, but trained instead to build on people's strengths. That is not to say a clinical psychologist or clinical social worker is incapable of doing these things. Clearly, some are, but that is based more on individual qualities of personality than anything else, because their training is more specialized on assessment and treatment. Therefore, we staffed this foundational level of entry to service with paraprofessional counsellors who specifically had that skill set.

Below is a condensed description of the program we developed in a partnership between South Shore Health and the South Shore Regional School Board. Please note that a comprehensive program description is not possible here, but this summary should at least demonstrate that what is described in this book is realistic and possible, and can cause dramatic improvements to the mental health and addiction system.

Structure of the Service

Tier 1

The health authority and school board were jointly involved in a number of health promotion initiatives. One program that is deserving of particular mention here is the full implementation of Promoting Alternative Thinking Strategies (SEAK, 2013). This program (PATHS) is an evidence-based, universal health promotion and prevention program demonstrated to prevent symptoms of anxiety and depression in children, among many other very significant outcomes. In our partnership, and with the assistance of others, we gradually expanded this program to all elementary schools in the region (to be completed Fall, 2016).

Tier 2

Each middle school and high school, on a weekly basis, had a community health worker (CHW) providing service on site. This was a paraprofessional, trained counsellor, employed by the mental health and addiction component of the health system. The primary function of that CHW was early-intervention counselling related to issues of addiction, mental health concerns, sexual health, and general life stresses and challenges. The amount of time spent providing this on-site counselling by the CHWs was determined by the population and service-demand at each school. This was adjusted regularly. At any point during the school year if it appeared that the client need was shifting, such that one school developed a higher demand, and another showed a reduction, staff schedules were readjusted to match. This needed to remain dynamic and ever-adjusting, and could not be rigid and static. Otherwise, it would not be client-centered.

Students could access their school-based CHW by contacting him/her directly to make an appointment, dropping-in (unscheduled) if the CHW was not with another student, or being referred from any school personnel (e.g., guidance counsellor, administrator, teacher). Each school also had a guidance counsellor (GC), employed by the school system. These were professionals trained to do traditional guidance work, but increasingly many of whom were also trained (and in some cases registered) as counselling therapists. They were able to provide most of the supports offered by the CHW, but also do more-therapeutic work in many cases. Students could access the GC directly for support, as another option if they chose not to see the CHW.

Having the CHW and the GC on site was intentional and was a significant benefit to the students/clients. It provided them with a wider array of skills to access and, more importantly, allowed them choice. Some students, because of an established trust with the GC, would be more comfortable accessing help there. Others, because of not wanting administration to know of their problems, may have chosen to access the CHW because he provides independent health service with different confidentiality rules. Having both roles in the school also allowed for very effective, day-to-day, collaborative care whenever possible.

Tier 3

A therapist (clinical social worker, clinical psychologist or counselling therapist) was assigned to collaborate with each school for therapy. These therapists were also based full time in the schools, and were employed by the mental health and addiction component of the health system. They collaborated with the CHW and GC to provide therapeutic interventions for clients deemed to require such a level of care. The therapist could not be accessed directly by students as an initial point of entry because, for most cases, it would not be the appropriate level of care (as previously discussed at length). Having students go first to a therapist would be the equivalent of a person with early signs of mildly increased blood pressure, going straight to a cardiovascular surgeon, when a family physician or nurse practitioner can assess and treat most such cases. The approach we took ensured we used the least-intrusive methods necessary to help the client, and also did not waste taxpayer dollars by over-serving clients.

A nurse practitioner or physician was assigned to collaborate with each CHW for sexual health services, such as exams or birth control prescriptions. The therapist or nurse practitioner was only engaged in a case by the CHW on an as-required basis. Because they provided more-specialized services, they were only used if that higher level of intervention (therapy or medical care) was actually needed.

Tier 4

A child and adolescent psychiatrist was available to see any clients deemed by any of the therapists to require medical/psychiatric care. Again, this was only if that higher level of intensity and intrusiveness was required.

Collaboration among Tiers

Each Tier 3 and 4 extended team member (therapist, nurse practitioner, psychiatrist) contributed collaboratively to the care of the client in whatever way worked best for the client. They could inform and advise one another in order to prevent clients from needing to see multiple people, or they could see the client jointly, separately, at school, out of school, with the GC, or perhaps with another agency involved. Whatever worked most efficiently and effectively *for the client* was what the team did. All of this work followed the principles of good integration and collaborative care described in this book.

Privacy and Confidentiality Between Schools and Health

This is a tricky topic, and the extent of complication is heavily dependent on the legislative environment in any particular jurisdiction. In Nova Scotia, there is no age of consent for health services. A young person can consent, independently of his parents, to engage in a health care service provided he is deemed competent to fully comprehend the nature of the service, and the risks and benefits associated with it. Therefore, in Nova Scotia, most young adolescents can be permitted to consent to the kind of early-intervention, supportive counselling, and therapy that was the foundation of this school-based service. He would be provided with a clear description of the service, and the inherent risks and benefits, which are all a normal part of the informed consent process anyway. If competent, and if he consented to this health care service, he would then be fully protected by privacy law. Even his parents or school principal would have no legal standing and no right to any information he shared in counselling, unless he gave permission.

From a client perspective, this was a great asset. It essentially placed all the power in his hands. It was client-centered. It allowed a student to access our services, knowing that he could share his most complicated or embarrassing thoughts or issues, and that even his parents would not be told (unless one of the exceptions to confidentiality occurs). Otherwise, he could access help safely.

While many parents find this issue of competency and no age of consent surprising and some openly disagree with it, it is, nonetheless, client-centered. This kind of legal framework eliminates a **very** significant barrier that keeps children and adolescents from seeking help. Many young people will avoid help if they believe their parents will need to be told or be involved in any way. As a parent, I can say unequivocally that I would rather my son be able to access help without my knowing, than to never get help at all because he needs my consent and doesn't want me to know.

The value of this kind of legislative framework cannot be overstated. In our experience, explaining these consent and privacy rules to an adolescent was empowering for them and made them more comfortable getting the help they needed. In jurisdictions that have a strict age of consent for health services, I would expect fewer young people to come forward for *early* help, but instead wait until it has escalated and parents or school staff notice and intervene. This is a systemic problem that is worth examining in such jurisdictions, as it is possibly the most significant barrier to access for adolescents.

Now, let's look at the privacy-related obligations of the schools. During the school day, the principal of the school is *in loco parentis*, which means she is in the role of parent while the child is at school that day. That means she has the responsibility to ensure the well-being of all the students. If she believes a student is facing any imminent or significant risk of any harm, she has an obligation to inform the parents. This is what makes for an interesting dynamic. It would appear that the health system must protect the information, while schools must share it. However, it is very possible to manage these dynamics if the education and health systems genuinely understand the need to be client-centered/student-centered, and do their best to disregard the traditional paternalism of the past in both systems.

Here are some of the key points of principle and action that we used in our program. When a youth was at school, he was in the care and control of the principal. When a student entered our health counselling service, he had done the same as if he walked across the street and entered his doctor's office or the hospital. He was at that moment protected under the health information privacy legislation that was in force. The health care provider had no independent legal right to share private information about any client with any school staff or administration, or with the youth's parents. The health care provider did have the right to seek permission from the student to share information with any particular person, and that student/client had the right to authorize or refuse such sharing. Most adolescent clients, once some initial rapport-building had happened, were comfortable allowing the counsellor to share and work collaboratively with parents or with certain trusted school staff, but it was still the client's decision.

The obligations of the health staff and the education staff regarding risk to self or others were pretty similar. If a student demonstrated that there was imminent and significant risk to herself (suicide), or risk to harm others, both sectors would be required to report this to the appropriate emergency services (911 for police or ambulance) for intervention to take place. However, the fact that a student had entered into a counselling process with someone from mental health and addictions did not mean the child was at risk, requiring the principal to report it to the parents. In a traditional, pathology-oriented program, staffed only by therapists, that may have been a reasonable conclusion. That was because in that traditional paradigm, in order even to be seen by a mental health clinician, the student would need to have demonstrated symptoms of a diagnosable condition. But, in a program that provides early support, counselling, coaching, and skill-building, in many cases there would be absolutely nothing to worry about. In fact, that's why we were doing it. Therefore, the fact that a student was seeing a mental health and addiction counsellor in school did not trigger the principal's obligation to report to the parent because it would not have been based on evidence of risk.

In any jurisdiction, if all of these issues are understood, discussed openly between the health and education partners, and focused entirely on making the systems fit the needs of students/clients, students can participate in education and participate in health services separately but within the same building. With consent, which is common, collaborative care can also take place. This is all simply contingent on the quality of the interagency partnership that is negotiated and developed, and the quality, creativity, flexibility, and client/student-centeredness of the leaders.

There is clearly more detail in this issue that cannot be fully explained here, and which will vary depending on the laws and policies in both health and education in any particular jurisdiction. The key point is that there should be a well-facilitated discussion that identifies those rules, and then finds all the possible ways to make services client-centered within the rules, or in spite of them. At the same time, any legislation or policies that inhibit good, comprehensive, client-centered care need to be challenged in an intentional and assertive manner. We all must play a role in that advocacy or nothing will change.

Results

As a result of this model being designed and implemented, our wait time for adolescents dropped from a high of five months down to 1-7 days. In other words, adolescents had same-day to same-week access. In addition, and somewhat ironically, we also dramatically increased the number of youth served. Over the first four years of this program, our numbers grew to the point of serving seven times as many adolescents per year as we had before this program. In terms of number of counselling and therapy sessions, in the fourth year we were providing 10 times as many sessions.

Actions for system managers and leaders:

1. Build an early-intervention support service in the schools, using paraprofessional counsellors, so the therapists can be used for those client who need and are waiting for therapy.

2. If your jurisdiction has an age of consent for health services, advocate for that to be eliminated, so young people can feel safe and comfortable getting help for their substance use, mental health, or sexual health concerns.

Actions for clients, supporters, and advocates:

1. Advocate actively for similar school-based services in your area. This approach has proven to increase access, and bring young people in who would never have gone to traditional, clinical or clinic-based services.

2. If your jurisdiction has an age of consent for health services, advocate for that to be eliminated, so young people can feel safe and comfortable getting help for their substance use, mental health, or sexual health concerns.

Creating a Single Team-Identity
Between Health and Education

One of the reasons why mental health and addiction staff were placed in the schools full time, without even having an office anywhere in the health authority, was to support their identification with school staff. We needed them to think of one another as co-workers, not as *us* and *them* (as per the concepts and methods explained at length in a previous chapter). From the beginning, staff of the mental health and addiction program were told to consider themselves to be part of the school staff. Reciprocally, school administrators, teachers and others were told to consider the health staff as part of the school team, not just visitors.

This approach helped build a sense that they were one team, with a single, collective job of helping to educate and care for the well-being of students. We also applied some of the other factors described earlier, which support the creation of that single-team identity. As we moved through the first year or two in this program, the walls between education staff and health staff eroded. In the majority of schools, that single-team identity in fact did develop. That is not to imply that staff members became unaware of their separate roles, employers, and skill sets. But, other than in a rare case or two, they reduced the *us/them* thinking that defined the past and prevented genuine collaboration.

This concept is obviously the same as trying to integrate mental health with addiction services. If we need to get two previously-separate groups of people to work and think as one, we must apply what we know about intergroup relations from social psychology. We must work to change their implicit and perhaps even unconscious definition of who is *us* and who is *them*. Again, this requires a great deal of work by leaders who can be flexible and abandon historical dogma about the separateness of mandates.

Example 2 – Withdrawal Management Services

As noted earlier, detox services in Nova Scotia had a history of over-serving clients with the most-intrusive approach possible – a hospital admission for all. As we worked to improve our ability to serve clients in a way that really fits their needs, we changed that. We converted our detox to a drop-in style program. One of the things we knew about many people with addictions is that when they are actively using, in crisis, and feeling desperate for help getting off their drug, they experience an incredible sense of urgency. However, most withdrawal management services in Nova Scotia required people to wait. They may have needed to wait because of limited availability of beds, or perhaps because of an administrative process for scheduling assessments and intakes. In any case, they did not always get the kind of help they needed, when they needed it.

People often get caught up in thinking the solution to a health problem is a specific place (detox unit), object (bed), or perhaps profession (doctor). What if the client were your brother? What is it that you would want available to him? It's simple. You would want help available, and the details would be less relevant. You would want to be able to take him somewhere right at the moment he expressed a genuine desire to get help. You would not want to wait for days or weeks while his motivation fades. You would want to be able to have some trained people start helping him today, in whatever program structure, place, or process was possible.

Based on this client-centered thinking, we converted our detox unit to a drop-in, day-program. Clients could simply come in and start working with staff on their withdrawal, without an appointment. The required medication orders were written by the physicians in the adjacent emergency department, thereby not requiring a dedicated physician to always be present. This was possible because we always recognized that we (Addiction and Mental Health Services, and the Emergency Department) were not separate, but rather were both part of one health care organization. The traditional walls between the programs were brought down. Clients could spend the day and evening being stabilized, resting, talking, and being monitored, but then could go home to sleep (least-intrusive method necessary) and come back in the morning. Clients who had completed the withdrawal process could continue to drop in as often as they wanted for ongoing work on relapse prevention. This was important because getting off the drug is not the hardest part, as anyone familiar with addiction knows. The biggest struggle is in learning to prevent relapse from that moment on. The program was completely responsive to the clients' needs.

This open model was designed more around that fact that very few people need hospitalization for withdrawal management, as withdrawal itself rarely poses a serious medical risk (except with alcohol). In our case, when a client did come along who clearly required 24-hour, medically-supervised withdrawal, arrangements would be made for admission to a hospital bed. But, that was uncommon. Our approach had been to design a service that provided for easy access and the least-intrusive care necessary to meet the needs of most people experiencing addiction issues. That required a flexible system that adapted constantly to *each* client, so that it would allow him in immediately and mold itself around his needs. Daily exceptions and customization of care became the norm. The service did not impose a one-size-fits-all approach just to achieve program standardization, because *it's not about us.*

Example 3 – Inpatient Mental Health Services

In our inpatient mental health services, we had a history of patients being kept for long periods of time, but not always with very active treatment. On occasion, some would go for as long as three or four days without seeing a psychiatrist. They would receive care from the nurses, of course, who would do an amazing job with great compassion and skill. But, the processes were not designed to actively and expediently treat the presenting illness so the person could be discharged and return to her home, family, and life. In addition, there was not a clear and comprehensive care plan developed upon admission to guide consistent work among all the staff. People knew the diagnosis, but a full plan was not documented.

This was yet another problem with processes, not staff. Again, we asked what it should be like if the client were our father or brother. Well, we would want a plan developed from the point of admission that addressed all aspects of his care (including *physical* health). All staff would be required to follow that plan consistently and could not stray from it unless agreed to by the treatment team. Every client would be seen by a psychiatrist at least once in every 24-48 hour period to continually reassess his condition, revise his treatment, and move him closer to being able to return home. We would want a community support worker on-site, dedicated to helping make plans for follow-up appointments, ensuring appropriate housing and support arrangements, developing life skills for independent living, etc. So, we did all those things, and improved the client-centeredness of the program. It made for more work in some ways for the staff and psychiatrist, but we merely kept remembering and reminding people that *it's not about us.*

Example 4 – Crisis Response Services

A crisis response service (CRS), in our rural area, is the service that responds primarily to the emergency department (ED) when a client arrives with acute and urgent mental illness issues. Before our transformation in the south shore of Nova Scotia, our CRS had some system-centered norms and processes. The staff were based at an office across town from the hospital. A call would come from the ED that a client was there in crisis and requiring assessment and appropriate treatment. The staff would find the client's file (if she had been a client before) and would take the time to review the whole chart.

The next step for the CRS nurse would be to head across town to the hospital and begin assessing the client. However, the traditional practice was to wait until the client was considered to be *medically cleared* by the ED. That meant no psychiatric assessment would start until the ED had completed all of its medical testing, received and interpreted all test results, and concluded there was no medical explanation for the presenting symptoms. That could take hours, depending on how busy the ED was, and what set of tests were ordered. After the client had waited (possibly for hours) in the ED waiting room, then waited (possibly for hours) in the exam room while medical tests were done, she would then need to start undergoing the psychiatric assessment process (possibly hours) by the CRS nurse and maybe psychiatrist. This *sequential* approach of waiting for medical clearance reflects the archaic conceptualization of a person consisting of two separate parts, the body and the mind.

But, wait... there's more. Depending on the staff member, if he was on lunch break when receiving a call, he might tell the ED that he would head over after lunch. Meanwhile, the staff of the ED would be struggling to manage a complex client who was rightfully the clinical responsibility of mental health and addictions, while also attending to the other patients requiring medical attention.

Our team asked the main question. If the client were our brother or daughter, how would I want this service to work? Well, we concluded, we would want the crisis team to be based at the hospital, so they are already right there in the building for faster response. So, we moved the staff. We would want the staff to respond immediately to the ED, and not spend a half hour reading the client's whole file. In the ED, doctors do not have the luxury of getting to read a patient's whole file before assessing the presenting symptoms. People would die if they did. Instead, they assess what is presented, and during the assessments and treatments they may consult the client's file for any issues directly relevant to the current/presenting symptoms. So, we stopped that in our process too. Staff would no longer take the time to read the whole file. Instead, they would just obtain the most-recent assessment and read that sometime *during* the work with the client, but they would not delay engaging with and assessing the client pending the reading of that information.

If the client were our brother, we would want him to be treated as a whole person, not as a body and a mind separately. Therefore, we eliminated the process of waiting for *medical clearance.* Instead, the CRS staff would start the assessment conversation with the client while the ED staff were also doing their medical work, and both would function collaboratively in the sharing of what they were observing. We would want a person who has shown up at the ED to be treated as having some urgency. This is both because he deserves it, and because to fail to do so would cause many other patients at the ED to wait longer than necessary while we block an exam room and drain staff time from other patients. Therefore, we implemented an expectation that CRS staff drop everything (yes, even their lunch) if called to the ED for a client in 'crisis'.

As a family member, we would also not want our distressed loved one to stay in the noise and uncomfortable chaos of an ED if not necessary. Therefore, we implemented a plan to bring the client out of the ED to an office downstairs in the mental health unit to conduct the psychiatric assessment. This made it a quieter, calmer, and a much more positive experience for the client and his family/friends who may have brought him in.

All the changes placed the client first, but also respected the fact that our delays negatively impacted on our ED colleagues' ability to do their very important and urgent medical work. We enhanced that understanding by working to integrate the CRS staff with the ED staff, and to create the same, singular-sense of group identity described several times in this book. We improved the client experience, improved the efficiency of the ED, improved interdepartmental collaboration, and all by simply focusing on the fact that *it's not about us.*

Example 5 – Sexual Assault Response Services

When the sexual assault response service was developed in the south shore of Nova Scotia, it accounted for all of the issues described in the chapter on early intervention. It was designed to be about the client, and about taking actions to prevent illness and maintain the survivor's mental health. It was also collectively designed by a number of people and community agencies, in an incredibly strong and high-functioning collaborative partnership.

Here is the way it worked within the health system component. When someone came to the hospital reporting an assault, two phone calls were made. One was to call in a trained sexual assault nurse examiner (SANE) and one to a mental health counsellor or therapist. Both came in immediately and began supporting the whole person. The counsellor was there for comfort, emotional support, trust-building, information, and linkage to mental health and addictions, as well as connections to any and all of the partnering community agencies that also provided supportive services.

By the time the medical care was provided, and the sexual assault exam was done, there was already rapport built with the counsellor, who could then offer immediate access to ongoing, supportive counselling or therapy. The intake team in the mental health and addiction program was directed and empowered to make any necessary adjustments to the master schedule in order to fit this survivor in as quickly as she wanted. That could include scheduling a clinician to work extra hours, or converting a clinician's administrative time to an appointment. The survivor would get an appointment as early as the same day or next day, unconditionally. She would not be put into a queue, and simply wait for an appointment weeks or months away. Because of the nature of the trauma, the risk of severe progression of mental illness as a result, and the great potential for prevention of that illness, this was given top priority.

In this program, the approach to the collection of evidence and the role of police, discussed earlier, was also considered critical. There were two detachments of the RCMP, as well as the Bridgewater Police Service, covering the jurisdiction, each responsible for some of the health district and some of the hospital sites. However, our previous establishment of high-functioning collaboration (like that described in this book), with the sole purpose of the client (survivor) being *the* priority, allowed an excellent system to develop among the multiple partners.

New forensic kits were kept at the hospitals. The sexual assault nurse examiners advised the client that if he chose to have the kit done, he would not be interviewed by police, and would not ever have to press charges if he didn't want to, but could choose to do so any time. Regardless of the location of the hospital involved, when an evidence kit was completed, the local police agency for that particular location (RCMP or municipal) was called to simply provide secure transport (for a tight chain of custody for the evidence), and all kits were brought to the Bridgewater Police Service for anonymous long-term storage. This inter-police collaboration meant the survivor maintained all the choice and power, had no police contact unless requested, and had a single, simple evidence-storage location for any time she might choose to proceed with charges. She would simply need to show up, provide some basic information, and the process would begin. Not only was it empowering, but it was also a simple, streamlined process for the client. This was all designed as a preventative approach to the potential worsening of the client's psychological experience.

This entire process was created by applying the depth of collaborative and client-centered partnerships described in this book. The genuine, collectivist approach taken by all the involved community agencies was nothing short of inspiring. Among the partners, the sophisticated and passionate understanding of client-centeredness at a system/process level was precedent-setting. At the time of writing this book, survivors of sexual assault in the south shore of Nova Scotia had the most client-centered and responsive services available in the province, especially in terms of preventative mental health support and care.

CHAPTER 14

CONCLUSIONS

Outpatient Work is the Backbone of the System

Much, but not all, of the focus of this book has been on improving the outpatient component of our programs. The primary reason is that it needs to function as the backbone or hub of the rest of the system. The vast majority of all people served in mental health and addiction programs are served on an outpatient basis, and that's even within the current, medical/psychiatric paradigm that only serves ill people. Imagine if we moved to a client-centered paradigm in which we served the even-larger number of people at the lower tiers who are not yet ill but simply need counselling and support to remain healthy.

Outpatient work is also the least intrusive, making it the most client-centered place to start. The stronger the outpatient services, the less often people will require inpatient admission because more of their needs will be met without such admissions. Also, the stronger and more comprehensive the outpatient services, the shorter the duration of inpatient care should be, when it is needed. This is simply because of our ability to provide the supportive follow-up and maintenance needed for people to be safely discharged.

The outpatient component of the system is the one that often receives the least attention and lowest priority, much like other areas of health care. There is a tendency, when working in a medical model, to ensure that the acute care work is never neglected, is always staffed and funded, and takes up much more management time than outpatient work. This is partly because the most-significant crises happen in that setting with the most-severely-ill people. It is also partly because, in a medical model, this acute care work is seen as requiring the highest level of expertise and specialization, thereby implying that it is the most important. This same reasoning also explains why, within outpatient services, the more intensive psychotherapy is the part of that gets the most attention and highest priority from the clinically-oriented leaders and managers.

Because of western cultural norms with regard to the dominance of the medical model, the public also often believes in the same unspoken hierarchy and professional elitism. People come to think that being admitted to a bed is good care and anything short of that is not. The circularity here is astonishing. We really only believe this because of the fact that we have a system that does not prevent our illnesses from getting worse. It waits until we are sick and treats our illness. In such a system, the health problems of many people have been permitted to worsen to the point that inpatient care is required far more often than necessary.

If we can start to make the switch to provide mental-health care, in addition to our current mental-illness care, we would see this begin to shift. People would start to realize that inpatient care is and should be the tiny part of the system way up at Tier 5, serving only a very small proportion of our people because most would be served earlier, thereby preventing serious illness from developing. People would start to see that the best care is the early outpatient care, and hospital admission is the last resort, which we should try to avoid.

Given the many points made in this book about the care being appropriate to the client's needs, and the value of early preventative work, it is clear that we need to build a robust, client-centered outpatient service that may be easily and quickly accessed and that places heavy emphasis on helping healthy people stay healthy. We need to maintain our ability to provide psychotherapy and psychiatric interventions, but *only* to those who can't be helped with less-intrusive methods.

Not a critique of the people

Please be clear that this book is not a critique of psychiatrists, psychologists, social workers, therapists, or administrators. The problems we are experiencing across Canada are caused by the system and the paradigm, not the people. Our problem is one of history and culture within that system. All of the people and professions are merely doing the job they were trained and hired to do. They are working within the norms of this field. They are simply seeing the programs, the clients, and the priorities the way they have been taught to see them.

I have met and known many hundreds of people who work in our public mental health and addiction field. With rare exception, the level of commitment to the well-being of the clients is outstanding. These people demonstrate compassion, selflessness, and professionalism. But, the system doesn't. Even though this book explicitly addresses the medical/psychiatric paradigm as a core target of change, this is not a reflection on the people in the medical profession. It is merely that those people are not always used in the right way for the right reasons within the system. We have clients being sent to psychiatrists who don't need a medical professional, and then, after we use their time so inappropriately, the psychiatrists get blamed for not being available enough for those really in need.

We have psychiatrists and therapists providing counselling, for which paraprofessionals would be more appropriate and cost-effective, and then, after we allow our most expensive resources to be used this way, we complain that we don't have enough resources. We have most other aspects of the system operating within that same medical model, even though the services in those areas are not medical and their clients do not require medical care. We have approaches to scheduling that are based on an historical, expert-centric model in which clients must contort their lives around the schedule of the psychologist, social worker, or other clinician. That is not the fault of these health care providers. It is just a legacy we have not yet changed.

We have a political climate in which providing illness care takes precedence over using evidence and policy to promote and create health because one can be done within an electoral term and referred to in campaigning, while the other requires long-term commitment to see the results. So, again, the pathology-oriented paradigm dominates in the end.

The people working in mental health and addictions are not the problem. The system that hires, connects, teaches, assimilates, guides, and directs those people is the problem. It is a system that was never actually *designed*. Instead, it has *evolved*, and has been incrementally tweaked over many decades, but was never intentionally constructed to be about the client. That is why the individual clients and our taxpaying public, when reflecting on the system and their place in it, commonly express the frustrating observation that *it's not about us, the clients.*

Going Forward – The Phenomenology of a Client-Centered System

The act of creating a client-centered system has no end point. There is no time when it is complete. It is an ongoing process of constantly asking the question *"What if the client was my loved one?"*. That question is the true test to use in this much-needed transformation. The medical/ psychiatric model on which our entire system is built approaches clients from an expert perspective. That is the nature of the model itself, and is entrenched because of such a lengthy history of that being normal, and being all that we know.

From one perspective, the shift being proposed in this book is one which is about systems, not people. Yet, from another perspective, it is about people. That is, it is about the way the policies, processes, and culture in our mental health and addiction programs actually *prevents* all the really good *people* in the system from doing the most client-centered work possible. So many staff working in these programs are empathic and compassionate individuals, who got into this field out of a genuine interest in helping people. When you work with these people, you see that. It is incredibly obvious and incredibly inspiring to see the level of engagement that so many show.

Unfortunately, all these staff must do their work according to the way the system and its programs are designed. They must follow procedures, work within policies, and deliver only the services that the program offers. This is very unfortunate, given that the nature of the program is determined by a paradigm that places expertise, illness-orientation, control, rigidity, paternalism, and system efficiency above the experience of the client. It is unfortunate that the paradigm is guided only by indicators and system-centric thinking, not by the feelings and subjective experiences of the clients. It is guided by a clinical orientation, rather than a client orientation.

We have a critically-important shift to make in all our mental health and addiction programs. It is a shift in the way we see the clients and the mandate of the program. We need to approach all our program decisions from the perspective of the client experience. We need to recognize that all members of the taxpaying public, not only those with disorders, are the clients. We need to listen to what they are saying. We need to build programs and processes that meet their needs (across the whole continuum). We need to engage in program transformation that puts the subjective experience of the clients first. We need to listen.

When a client or advocate is expressing concerns to the media, we need to avoid hearing *another complaint*. Instead, we must listen to what the theme is. It is simple. When our public talks about the mental health and addiction programs and how they work, they are clearly and simply saying *it's not about us*. It's about politics, money, administrators trying to run a tight ship, data collection, clinical expertise, schedules that are convenient for staff, etc.,… but *it's not about us*, the clients and the public.

It is time for that to change. It is time that those running the programs start to do so from the client perspective. It is time to stop saying that programs and organizations are client-centered, while still making decisions and building processes that favour the needs of the system over those of the client. Such hypocrisy is no longer being tolerated by the public. It is time to see the world through the eyes of the client, and make their needs the real priority, which requires sacrificing some of the typical needs of the system, moving away from the expert-driven way of serving people, and building empathy into administration. The health care providers have empathy. The culture of administration does not. People in administration are focused on the things that their culture emphasizes and reinforces, because that is the job.

But, what if a few administrators started imagining their mother, their son, or their sister as the client? What if they then made policy, system, program, staffing, and structure decisions based on what they would want their dad's experience to be? What if their decisions were made to create the kind of service that could help *prevent* their brother from ever needing a diagnosis of mental illness or a hospital bed?

I believe that we can get to a place where our public is healthy; where people feel supported in their workplaces and schools to stay healthy; where people can be helped with conversations and skill-building when they begin to struggle; and where people can still also receive psychotherapy and psychiatric intervention if and when their problems escalate to that point. I believe we can get to a point where *every* level of support and care provided is quickly accessible and is available right where people live, study, work, shop, or receive other health care services. I believe we can reach a point where governments will start strategically and courageously using public policy to ensure the mental health of the next generation, and prevent people from developing addictions or mental illness.

This move from a system-centered, pathology-oriented, medical/psychiatric model to a client-centered paradigm is the secret to transforming our system in Canada. To get started, it merely requires a change in perspective. We must get out of our own egocentric tendencies and work hard to understand the unique, diverse, and essential subjective experience of the client. We need to start understanding that empathy and client-centeredness are not only clinical concepts, but are vital tools for administrators and leaders if we hope to ever make real change in our systems. What if the client were your daughter? Simply put, within the mental health and addiction system, leaders must start to recognize and repeatedly remind themselves and staff that *it's not about us*…it's about the client.

Final actions for clients, supporters, and advocates:

Those of you who have had negative experiences with this system across Canada, this is an opportunity to lead real change. Your voice is incredibly powerful. Your experiences are extremely insightful and useful. Be an advocate for this change. Talk or write to the elected officials in your province, or at the federal level. Talk or write to the CEO, vice presidents, directors, and managers of your local health system and mental health and addiction program. Talk or write to the media. Tell them it's time for the system to be about the client. Tell them we need to make this shift from the medical model to a client-centered paradigm. Tell them to follow the simple processes described in this book, by asking the most important question…if the client was you brother, sister, mother, father, spouse, child, grandparent, etc., how would you want this system to work. Use this book as a tool to help guide the shift to this new way of thinking about **system design**.

Whatever you do, remember that if nobody advocates for this, we are guaranteed to never get it. A friend of mine used to paraphrase Wayne Gretzky when my daughter was playing basketball as a child, by telling her "you miss every shot you don't take". So, if we don't advocate for this change, there is no reason to expect it to happen. Your voice matters, even as only one person, because it will spark others to also use their voices. Famous anthropologist Margaret Mead is responsible for my favourite quote of all time… "Never doubt that a small group of thoughtful, committed citizens can change the world; indeed, it's the only thing that ever has.". The biggest changes in our world, from women being allowed to vote in Canada, to legalization of same-sex marriage, to abolishment of apartheid in South Africa, all started with one person saying *'this is wrong, and we should change it'*. Then someone else heard that and said *'I agree, this is wrong and we should change* it'. The next thing you know we have the million-man march, the abolishment of slavery, or the overthrowing of an oppressive dictatorship. In all cases, it started with one person like you. **Be that voice.**

Final actions for system managers and leaders:

Those who have been, are presently, or will be program leaders or people of influence over the mental health and addiction system must start to recognize and repeatedly remind ourselves and staff what our jobs are really supposed to be about. In terms of their core purpose, they are not supposed to be about the staff, the history, the system's efficiency, the unions, the manager's need for control, the leaders' desire for complete standardization, the academic need for data collection, the protection of turf, or maintaining professional elitism. They also are not supposed to be about only delivering the kinds of services most of our clinically-oriented program leaders and staff happen to understand, prefer, and be comfortable with, which is treating people *after* they are already ill. All of those things are our issues, our biases, our preferences, our professional blind-spots and limitations, our insecurities, our attachment to the past, and our dogma. It is time to become more self-aware and abandon all of these things that are our own issues, and create a system that is about the client instead because... *it's not about us!*

REFERENCES

Armstrong, L. (2015, May 5). Ontario youth wait a year or more for mental health care: report. *Toronto Star.* Retrieved from https://www.thestar.com

Babor, T. F., Caetano, R., Casswell, S., Edwards, G., & Geisbrecht, N. (2010). *Alcohol: No ordinary commodity: Research and public policy.* Oxford: Oxford University Press.

Bird, H. (2015, April 29). N.W.T.'s mental health care system failed our son, say grieving parents. *CBC News North.* Retrieved from http://www.cbc.ca

Canadian Centre on Substance Abuse. (2015). *Cannabis regulation: Lessons learned in Colorado and Washington State* (National Release of Report on Marijuana). Retrieved from Canadian Centre on Substance Abuse website: http://www.ccsa.ca/Resource%20Library/CCSA-Cannabis-Regulation-Lessons-Learned-Report-2015-en.pdf

CBC News. (2010, April 12). Mental health system failing, says Calgary widow. *CBC News Calgary.* Retrieved from http://www.cbc.ca/news/canada/calgary/mental-health-system-failing-says-calgary-widow-1.924763

CBC News. (2013, April 9). B.C. mental health system failing teens, watchdog says. *CBC News British Columbia.* Retrieved from http://

www.cbc.ca/news/canada/british-columbia/b-c-mental-health-system-failing-teens-watchdog-says-1.1330994

CBC News. (2014, April 10). Case exposes failings of mental health system: lawyer. *CBC News Newfoundland & Labrador.* Retrieved from http://www.cbc.ca/news/canada/newfoundland-labrador/case-exposes-failings-of-mental-health-system-lawyer-1.2605999

CBC News. (2014, December 30). Mental-health help for youth needs radical reform, says advocate Tony Boeckh. *CBC News Montreal.* Retrieved from http://www.cbc.ca

Colwell, S. (2013, October 29). Wait times reduced by months for mental health, addictions help. *Lighthouse Now.* Retrieved from http://leader-development.ca/sites/default/files/2013-10-29%20Lighthouse%20-%20Wait%20times%20reduced%20by%20months%20for%20mental%20health%2C%20addictions%20help.pdf

Colwell, S. (2014, March 4). Student access to health services shows dramatic improvement. *Lighthouse Now.* Retrieved from http://leader-development.ca/sites/default/files/2014-03-04%20Lighthouse%20-%20Student%20access%20to%20health%20services%20shows%20dramatic%20improvement.pdf

Corcoran, K. (2012, October 10). Health services expand at South Shore schools. *Lighthouse Now.* Retrieved from http://leader-development.ca/sites/default/files/2012-10-10%20Lighthouse%20-%20Health%20services%20expand%20at%20South%20Shore%20schools.pdf

Coubrough, J. (2016, February 1). Discharged: Mental health patients raise alarms about care in Winnipeg. *CBC News Manitoba.* Retrieved from http://www.cbc.ca

Crépault, J. (2014). *Cannabis policy framework.* Retrieved from Centre for Addiction and Mental Health website: https://www.camh.ca/en/hospital/about_camh/influencing_public_policy/Documents/CAMHCannabisPolicyFramework.pdf

Day, J. (2014, January 9). Province urged to act on Prince Edward Island mental health crisis. *The Guardian.* Retrieved from http://www. theguardian.pe.ca/News/Local/2014-01-09/article-3569475/ Province-urged-to-act-on-Prince-Edward-Island-mental-health- crisis/1

Embry, D. (2016). PAX Good Behaviour Game. *Paxis Institute.* Retrieved from http://goodbehaviorgame.org/

Henton, D. (2015, December 7). Mental health review will show fragmented system, failures to act on previous recommendations: Swann. *Calgary Herald.* Retrieved from http://calgaryherald.com

Herie, M., & Skinner, W. W. (2014). *Fundamentals of addiction: A practical guide for counsellors* (4th ed.). Toronto, Canada: Centre for Addiction and Mental Health.

Heroux, D. (2016, April 3). Sask. mom wants quicker access to mental health consultant after son dies from fentanyl overdose. *CBC News Saskatoon.* Retrieved from http://www.cbc.ca

Hounsell, K. (2016, April 19). N.S. woman struggling to find mental health services for friend in need. *CTV News Atlantic.* Retrieved from http://atlantic.ctvnews.ca/n-s-woman-struggling-to-find-mental- health-services-for-friend-in-need-1.2865967

Kingsbury, S., & York, A. (2013). *The choice and partnership approach.* Retrieved from http://www.capa.co.uk/

Kirby, M. (2013, October 7). We are failing young Canadians on mental health. *Toronto Star.* Retrieved from https://www.thestar.com

Kitts-Goguen, C. (2015, October 29). Wait times for mental health referrals longest in central N.B. *CBC News New Brunswick.* Retrieved from http://www.cbc.ca

LeBlanc-Smith, Y. (2015, November 5). Cape Breton mother wants mental health inquiry after son's death. *CBC News Nova Scotia.* Retrieved from http://www.cbc.ca

Lee, M. (2016, January 27). Big gains for mental health in South Shore. *Lighthouse Now.* Retrieved from https://lighthousenow.ca/article.php?title=Big_gains_for_mental_health_in_South_Shore

Meichenbaum, D., & Turk, D. C. (1987). *Facilitating treatment adherence: A practitioner's guidebook.* New York, NY: Plenum Press.

Ricci, T. (2016, April 5). Winnipeg mom calling for change in Manitoba's mental health system. *Global News BC.* Retrieved from http://globalnews.ca

Rush, B. (2010). *Tiered frameworks for planning substance use service delivery systems: Origins and key principles* (CAMH Report Vol. 27). Retrieved from Nordic Studies on Alcohol and Drugs website: http://www.nordic http://www.nordicwelfare.org/PageFiles/4930/08_Rush.pdf

Scott, S. (2016, April 14). Yellowknife LGBTQ community wants more inclusive health care system. *CBC News North.* Retrieved from http://www.cbc.ca

Socially and Emotionally Aware Kids (SEAK) Project. (2013). *PATHS findings from phase II.* Retrieved from http://seakproject.com/current-findings/

Taweel, H. (2016, February 18). Critical gaps exist in mental health services in P.E.I. for vulnerable children, youth. *The Guardian.* Retrieved from http://www.theguardian.pe.ca/News/Local/2016-02-18/article-4439935/Critical-gaps-exist-in-mental-health-services-in-P.E.I.-for-vulnerable-children,-youth/1

The Chronicle Herald. (2016, January 14). Mental health services harder to reach in Nova Scotia. *The Chronicle Herald.* Retrieved from http://thechronicleherald.ca

Thomson, N. (2016, March 14). Ross River, Yukon, residents desperate for mental health services. *CBC News North.* Retrieved from http://www.cbc.ca

Ubelacker, S. (2016, February 3). Young people often forced to seek help for mental health issues at ER, study says. *CBC News Toronto.* Retrieved from http://www.cbc.ca

University of Waterloo, School of Public Health and Health Systems. (2015). *Canada's mental health system is failing children in crisis.* Retrieved from https://uwaterloo.ca/public-health-and-health-systems/canadas-mental-health-system-failing-children-crisis

Ware, B. (2013, October 21). South Shore wait times slashed; Mental health, addiction services take 4 weeks instead of 8 months. *The Chronicle Herald.* Retrieved from http://thechronicleherald.ca

Ware, B. (2014, February 17). South Shore students' mental health wait times cut. *The Chronicle Herald.* Retrieved from http://thechronicleherald.ca

Weber, B. (2013, June 5). Suicide study reveals depth of Nunavut's mental health problems. *The Globe and Mail.* Retrieved from http://www.theglobeandmail.com

ACKNOWLEDGEMENTS

It is essential to note that the accomplishments and system transformations described in this book are the result of hard work by the most effective leadership team with whom I have ever worked. They include Janet Sears, Clara Miller, Brent Laybolt, Yvonne DaSilva, Jeannie Chisholm, Kelly Becker, and Dr. Andrew Ashley-Smith. It was a true honour to get to work collaboratively with this incredibly talented, intelligent, passionate, and courageous team of leaders. Thank you.

What I know about principle-centered leadership, I learned from my mentor, long-time colleague, editor, and friend, Hubert Devine. Thank you for your steadfast wisdom.

I must acknowledge the amazing commitment to building a client-centered system that was demonstrated by the wonderful staff of the Addiction and Mental Health program of the former South Shore Health in Nova Scotia. Their faith in the vision, their tolerance for uncertainty and ambiguity as we cut a new path through this forest, and their willingness to both trust and *challenge* me and the leadership team to ensure we made the best decisions for the clients was deeply inspiring. I appreciated and enjoyed *every single assertive debate*. Thank you.

During this program transformation, none of these changes would have been possible without the unconditional trust and support provided by CEO, Dr. Peter Vaughan, and Vice President, Janet Simm. They are the embodiment of empowering leadership. Thank you.

The truly remarkable level of integration of support and treatment services into the school system, and the extraordinary depth of partnership between South Shore Health and the South Shore Regional School Board was made possible by several key people. It would never have evolved and thrived as it did without the initial creativity and vision of Kari Barkhouse, and the unwavering commitment to collaborative and student-centered decision-making demonstrated by Steve Prest, Nancy Pynch-Worthylake, Jeff DeWolfe, Darren Haley, and Mark MacLeod. It also would never have happened without the genuineness, flexibility, and collaborative skills shown by the many staff, guidance counsellors, and administrators in all the schools in the region. Thank you.

The partnership between health and police was also remarkable, and contributed greatly to the progress on which this book is based. Those leaders include John Collyer and Scott Feener of the Bridgewater Police Service, and Jean-Guy Richard, Derek Smith, Paul McDougall, and Sandi Merrill of the RCMP in Lunenburg and Queens Counties. Thank you.

Thanks are owed to my co-founders of the Sexual Assault Services of Lunenburg and Queens, which included Coordinators Stacey Godsoe and Diane Crowell, Lynn Farrell and Donna Crouse (with the former South Shore Health), the policing leaders named in the paragraph above, Jeanne Fay (Second Story Women's Centre), recently-retired Katherine McCarron (Harbour House), Julie Veinot (Sexual Health Centre of Lunenburg County), and Karen Crofton (Provincial Victim Services Program). In addition, I thank Art Fisher of the Family Services Association of Western Nova Scotia for his leadership of various collaborative partnerships, and for never allowing his thinking (or mine) to be contained inside any box. Thank you all.

A number of other generous people directly contributed to, or assisted in, the construction of this book. Those include Cindy Zinck (without whose contribution the book would not have been written), Shauna Davies, Jack Davies, Sara Ramsay, Miranda Veinot, Brittany Cormier, Marguerite MacDonald, and Shelly Shea. Also a special thanks to Kenzie Butt, who selflessly contributed her outstanding intelligence, insights, principles, and wisdom throughout the writing of the book, and provided irreplaceable and continuous inspiration. Thank you all.

Thank you to my dear friend, Wendy Black, and the Around the Bend Foundation, for always believing in the principles of client-centered service, and for being a constant source of motivation to make a real difference in the lives of our youth.

Thanks to the thousands of psychology students at Saint Mary's University, from whom I have learned many important life lessons, and who never fail to inspire me with their passion for improving the world and the lives of the people around them. Thank you.

Thanks to the loves of my life – my wonderful wife of 28 years, Alma, and my amazing son and daughter, Brian and Ali, for consistently (though perhaps unknowingly) keeping me inspired to make a positive contribution to the world. Also, thanks to my parents, Brian Leader and Alda Swain, for giving me a passion for social justice and the confidence to constantly challenge the systems that get in its way. Thank you.

Finally, and most importantly, my sincere thanks to all the clients, family members, and advocates, who have directly or indirectly provided feedback (positive and negative) and advice on how to do it better. For those who directly shared your concerns with me about programs under my leadership, those of you across this country who have expressed your frustrations through the media and online, and all those who have actively advocated for system change anywhere in Canada, this book is fully anchored in the insights and experiences you have been courageous enough to share. THANK YOU!

ABOUT THE AUTHOR

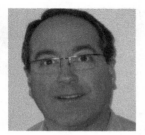 Todd Leader is a psychologist and a social worker who has spent the last 26 years leading health service development and transformation, as well as health promotion, particularly in the areas of mental health, addictions, and primary health care. He has also been teaching in the Faculty of Science at Saint Mary's University for the same 26 years. Todd has earned the Excellence in Teaching Award from the Saint Mary's University Students' Association, and health services under his leadership have earned two international best practice awards, and a leadership award for excellence in women's health. He has been the President of the Public Health Association of Nova Scotia and a member of the Board of Directors of the Canadian Public Health Association. Todd has been consulted by the Canadian Centre of Substance Abuse regarding integration of mental health and addictions. At the time of writing this book, he was also the President-Elect of the Association of Psychologists of Nova Scotia. Most recently, he was appointed by the Nova Scotia Minister of Health and Wellness to the Ministerial Panel on Innovation in Mental Health and Addictions. Todd has spent his whole career working as an advocate for evidence-based, client- and community-centered programs, systems, and public policy. This book is the result of that experience.

CONNECT WITH ME

Facebook: https://www.facebook.com/todd.leaderdevelopment/

Twitter: @toddleader1

Linkedin: https://ca.linkedin.com/in/toddleaderdevelopment

Cathydia Press Website: www.cathydiapress.ca

CPSIA information can be obtained
at www.ICGtesting.com
Printed in the USA
LVHW02s1927180818
587386LV00003B/567/P